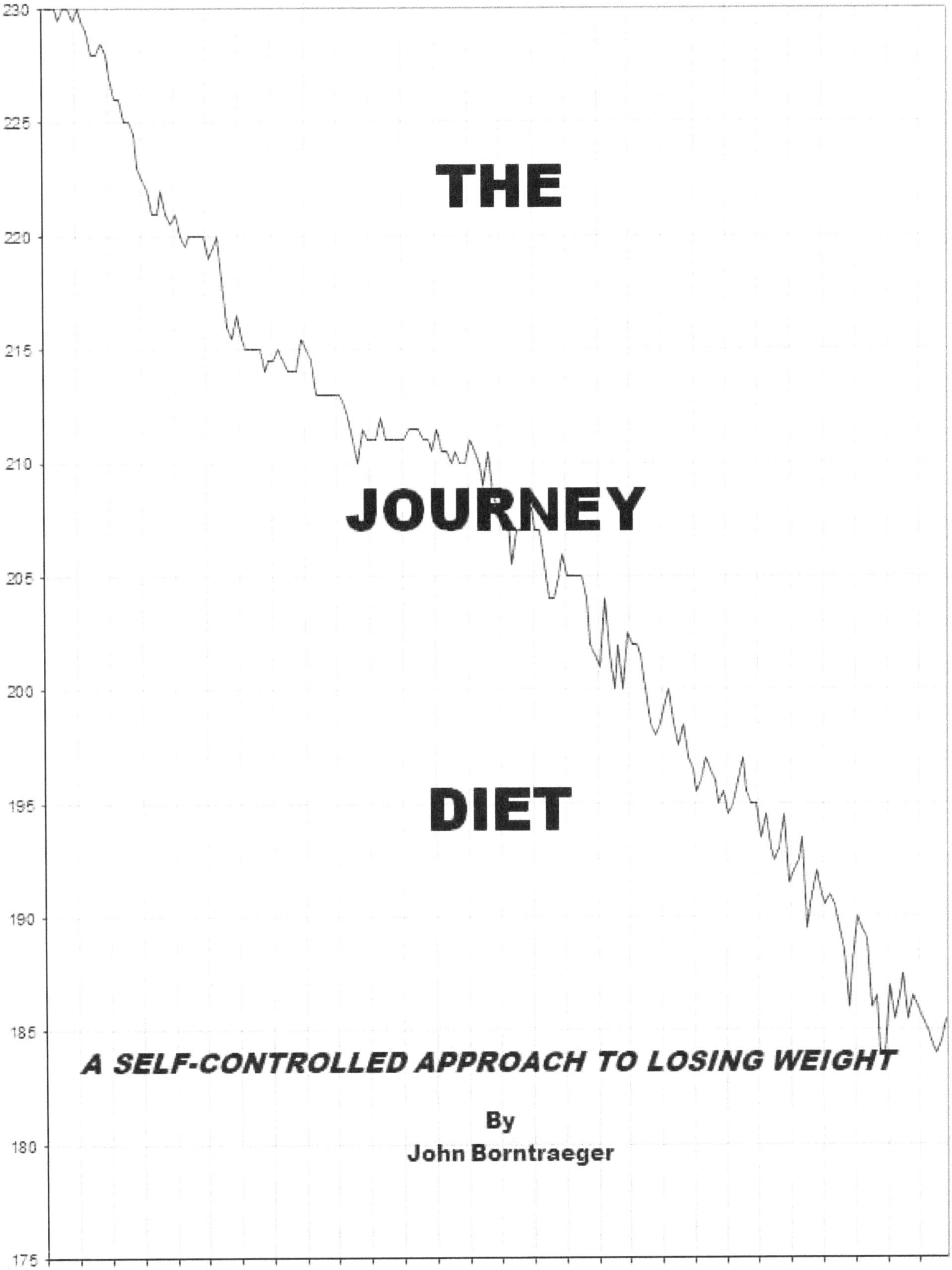

THE

JOURNEY

DIET

A SELF-CONTROLLED APPROACH TO LOSING WEIGHT

By

John Borntraeger

John Borntraeger

Copyright 2018 by John Borntraeger

The Journey Diet by John Borntraeger

ISBN 9-781-79577099-6

https://www.thejourneydiet.com

To

Christina & Eddie

They are

The Stars in My Sky

And To

My Grace Mary

She Is

The Healer of My Heart

And

The Love of My Life

CONTENTS

Acknowledgements

I would like to give thanks to those who assisted in the writing of this book. The friends listed here not only found multiple grammatical errors in reading this text over and over again, but also gave opinions concerning the content, both supportive and critical. I am especially indebted to those whose advice resulted in emphasis of, and more thorough explanation of, the multiple health aspects of this process. Their input resulted in vast improvements of the text and assisted in assuring the reader is aware of the importance of the many aspects of this weight-loss and health improvement process.

Whether it was giving opinions as to accuracy of text or just proof-reading, or both, I am indebted to Grace Borntraeger, Bonnie Chester, Amy Wixted, MPH, CHES, CIC; Robert Reilly MD, FACP; Jill Miller, RN, CDE; and Kristen Curtis MS RD LDN.

INTRODUCTION

You know, the important word in the title of this book is "Journey" and not "diet." And to be truthful, I really don't like the title of this book. Though the title says it's a diet, I don't think of it as a diet. At least I don't think it's a diet anyway similar to those with which we are familiar. But if the title were <u>The Journey</u>, you would never know it's about losing weight.

I wanted the title to be, "It's Not Really A Diet Book." And when I started writing it in 1974 that was the title and it remained the title until I retired in 2009 and had the time to finish the book. "Why that title?" you ask. Well, as I said, this really is about diet. But it is not a "diet" in the sense that most of us think of when we hear that word. Most people hear the word diet and they immediately conjure up images of pain, denial, eating things they can't stand, not eating the things they love, sweating at the gym, doing things they've never done before, and usually, they think of these horrible times extended over months and months. And then, as is usually the case, the weight will be back as soon as the dieter returns to his or her normal life style. Let's be honest. No one really wants to live a life of denial, eating food they can't stand. Eating is one of the greatest gifts in life. After all, how do we celebrate an anniversary? We go out and have a fine dinner. And, how do parents reward a child for good deed? Quite often, it's done with a treat. And hopefully, it's ice cream. It is unfortunate that the word diet brings about all of these negative images. It really shouldn't.

The word diet refers to the food we eat. If we live on fast food, or we eat vegetarian meals, that is our diet. The key word here is "ON." What we eat IS our diet. However, if we are "ON" a diet, then immediately, a different and often miserable way of life is suddenly imagined. If you were to meet an old friend and he said to you, "I'm on a diet," you would immediately look at his waist. Why? To see how big he is. If he said to you, "I'm a vegetarian," you would not think to yourself, "Ah, he's on a diet." But he is! He's not just "ON" a diet. Eating vegetarian "IS" his diet. So, don't think of the journey you are about to begin as being "ON" a diet. Think about this journey as a very slow and pleasant way of changing your lifestyle. It's a journey with a destination of an improved lifestyle. And your diet (that is what you eat) is a very important part of that lifestyle. If you think of this as being "ON" a diet, then you must also think about what's going to happen when you finish and you get "OFF" the diet. The difference here is that when you finish this journey, you will not change what you eat (your diet). Therefore, you were not ON a diet. You merely taught yourself to modify the foods you eat (your diet) and to modify your lifestyle for a more healthy future. Yes, we are going to talk a great deal about your diet. But we (actually you) are going to take a journey to modify your lifestyle. So even though you will not be ON a diet, as most would define it, we will still call this "The Journey Diet."

So you see using the word "ON" implies that you're going to <u>change</u> your eating habits to something that is different or abnormal. And these eating habits will last only as long as the diet. And when the diet is over, the eating habits of "the diet" will end. So the mental image formed about a diet is that the person is no longer going to eat the "normal" way, or eat a "normal" diet. He or she is going to undertake an abnormal eating routine. It is true that the person undertaking this journey will no longer eat the way he or she did previously. And that's good, because the person's diet is probably a contributing factor to his or her overweight condition. The issue here is that this process is far from abnormal. It is simply a process where a simple self-taught routine is developed and the person learns to live an improved lifestyle, which of course includes improved eating habits. In the first paragraph there is a sentence that stated, "And then, as is usually the case, the weight will be back as soon as the dieter returns to his or her normal life style." Why do you think so many people lose weight on diets and then gain it all back? The answer is that their "diet" didn't prepare them for their life "after" the diet. That's the difference between being on a diet and undertaking the journey described here.

This book then does deal with a diet: your diet. But it is not a program to lose all kinds of weight by denying yourself of the things you love. That simply will not work! And even if losing weight through denial does work for you, chances are that as soon as you return to your "normal" life style, a life style you're comfortable with, the weight will come right back. The key here is that a denial type of dieting doesn't help you change your lifestyle for the long term.

So, as you begin this journey to change the way you live, remember there are no demands that you give up the things you love. You may eventually give them up. But that will be a decision <u>you</u> make. Other food items you won't give up. But you will eat less of them and eat them less often. And you will decide when and how much you eat of these items. And that decision will be based upon all the lessons you will learn about yourself and your weight. And these are lessons you will teach yourself on this journey. But again, what you eat and how much will be your choice. But it will be an intelligent choice. And these choices will be based upon your experiences. This journey can result in your being in charge of your diet (the food you eat). And it can result in a significant weight loss and a much healthier lifestyle that results in keeping the excess weight off.

So, let's get started.

John Borntraeger

Chapter 1

MENTAL ATTITUDE

It is very, very difficult to change your attitude toward something. And, as mentioned before, we all have a negative attitude toward dieting. And it is this negative attitude that quite often spells doom to an effort to lose weight.

Attitude is probably the most important factor when an individual undertakes a change in lifestyle. The attitude issue was indirectly touched upon in the introduction where it was stated, "And then, as is usually the case, the weight will be back as soon as the dieter returns to his or her normal life style." With this type of attitude it's an absolute certainty the lost weight will find its way back. In fact, with this attitude, there's a good chance your journey will not take you very far in the lifestyle change that is probably needed.

Let's face one fact. If we go into a diet with the attitude, "this isn't going to work," I guarantee it won't. The success of an effort to lose weight is very much dependent upon our attitude. Therefore, when we think of the word "diet," along with it comes all the negative images, our attitude suffers, and so does the chance of success. Think for a moment about two baseball players going to the plate to bat. They will be facing a pitcher who has struck out both of them in their two previous times at bat. The first one thinks to himself, "This guy has already struck me out two times. I don't stand a chance of getting a hit. I'm just wasting my time trying to get a hit off this guy." The second player goes to the plate with a positive attitude, thinking to himself, "Okay. This pitcher got lucky the first two times. This time I get even. I'm gonna smack that ball so far they'll never find it." Which player do you think has a better chance of getting a hit?

So, you can begin this process with the attitude that you're going to successfully change your lifestyle; to live better and longer.   Or, you can begin this journey, probably a very short journey, with the attitude that "I can't do this." "I'll always be heavy." "I just don't have any will-power." The choice is yours. And believe me, IT IS A CHOICE!

So, you must understand and believe that dieting is first of all, a mental thing. And to help with this attitude change, we will no longer call our effort "A DIET". And you shouldn't either. Whatever you do, don't tell anyone you're on a diet. Because you're not! You are making an effort to change your lifestyle! You are going to make some changes <u>to</u> your "diet," and quite possibly change some other aspects of your lifestyle. But you are **NOT ON A DIET**! What should you say to someone who notices you have slimmed down a bit? It's simple. Just tell them the truth. Tell them, "Well, yes I have lost a few pounds." "And I've done it by just eating more intelligently." "I'm eating smarter and getting a little more active." And it's the truth. You don't have to eat all the strange concoctions you find in the various diet cook-books and run 2 miles every night. And you don't have to wait for the mailman or the UPS guy to bring tomorrow's breakfast to your front door. And notice I said, "… a little more active." I didn't use the word "exercise." You'll find out later that I hate that word and all the connotations associated with it.

You are going to determine what foods negatively affect your weight and your physical well-being. You are also going to learn how the quantities of food can negatively affect your weight and your physical well-being. In addition, you are going to find out how physical activity can affect your weight. This will be a self-teaching activity. It has to be. Not everyone burns the same amount of calories for a given activity. There are some who can eat twice as much as I, and yet are very slim. They could eat a half- dozen doughnuts and not gain an ounce. If I as much as look at one of those doughnuts, I'll gain three pounds.

Did you catch the negative attitude here? We all know that it's impossible to gain weight just by looking at food. Yet, we think of ourselves that way. We think, "poor me, I'll gain weight no matter how hard I try." Baloney! If we weigh more than we should, for our own well-being, we must learn why. Then slowly change our living habits. There are two key words here: SLOWLY and LIVING. I didn't say to change our eating habits. I said to change our living habits. This of course includes eating. But it is a great deal more than just eating.

The second key word is SLOWLY. A quick weight loss is not healthy. The chances are that a rapid weight loss will be at the expense of your physical well-being. In fact, there have been reports about people having very serious health problems due to rapid weight loss. There may have been other circumstances that play a part in these medical problems associated with dieting, but the point is that rapid weight loss is unhealthy. And you probably can't or won't want to continue the lifestyle that brought about this rapid weight loss. Very few of us gained the weight rapidly. So why would we expect to lose it rapidly. It probably took many years to put on that extra weight. We usually form poor lifestyle habits very slowly. So, to try and change our body weight or to change our eating habits very rapidly is utterly stupid and dangerous. And the chances are pretty good the weight will not stay off. And, while we are on the health aspects of changing our life style, anyone, including you, should consult your physician before trying to lose weight, either through changing eating habits or through increased physical activity, or both. A good physical exam is never a waste of money. In fact, it quite often helps in the improved mental attitude you must have to successfully change your life style. So, visit your physician. Tell him or her how you plan to change your eating habits, and what physical activities you plan to undertake. And, during this experience keep in contact with your doctor to have him or her monitor your health.

The mental attitude we have affects everything we do. If we think of some sad occurrence in our life, it is sometimes difficult to get ourselves out of the "blues." That is why you must not think of this as a diet. It isn't. You're not going to have to give up the foods you love. What you will do, if you have the right mental attitude, is to teach yourself to limit the quantities. At some point, you'll convince yourself that you don't want that second piece of cake. And quite possibly you will begin to think, "I don't even want the first piece of cake." And that my friend, is not denial. That is intelligent eating. It is <u>not</u> something I tell you that you must do. It is something <u>you</u> choose to do. When you reach that point, and you will, you have placed yourself in control. You could eat the piece of cake if you wanted to. But you'll find you don't want it. You will find that there is nothing wrong with having a piece of cake. And occasionally you will, knowing that you are in control, have a piece of that delicious cake. But having two pieces at every meal is catastrophic. You will learn this and you will not even think of having the second piece.

And you will find that it is really easy to get to the point where you are in control. There is only one requirement. And I can hear you now. Oh Boy! Here it comes. Here's the catch. What do I have to do? Actually, you don't to do much at this stage, except to decide that you DO want to change your personal appearance and very probably, your health. It requires a commitment on your part. That's all. A firm commitment that "I can and will change my life style (eating habits, and activity habits, if necessary) and lose the weight I want to lose." We'll talk more about commitment a bit later. For now, we'll just say that your commitment drives the attitude. And your ATTITUDE is critical to the success of your effort.

As a high school senior, I attended a college night where I met the dean of the university I hoped to attend. I will never, ever forget his words that night. He said, "There is nothing in this world that can help you get through my school, except the shear determination to do it. No matter how smart you are, if you don't want it bad enough, you won't make it." And believe me, he was right. There were many, many times during my years in college I thought of his words and it was, in fact, those very words that helped get me through and graduate. It was a hard five years and many people, much smarter than I, fell by the wayside. And it is the same with this process of changing your lifestyle to slim down, and promote better health, and a longer life. Following this process to a much healthier lifestyle will succeed for you, only if you want it bad enough.

In addition, you must understand that the techniques you are going to teach yourself will take time. This is not a quick weight loss process. That is not the intention. For some, however, the weight loss can be quite rapid. Personally, I think it has a little to do with the right mental attitude. It's like anything else in life. The harder you try, the better, and sometimes, the quicker the results come about. But it is also due to the fact that each of us burn calories at different rates. And, you will find that as you get older, it seems you burn fewer calories for a given activity than when you were young. That is why is it so important that you learn to maintain, through good living habits, a good body weight before you get too old. It is much more difficult for older folks to shed weight through activity. It is also a little more difficult to change your eating habits as you get older. Unfortunate, isn't it?

It does take time, and here lies the one problem you must overcome. That positive mental attitude begins to weaken the longer it takes to begin seeing results. Many of us have made a New Year's resolution to lose weight, only to give up on the effort because we didn't lose 5 pounds by January 5th. And, as I mentioned before, most diets are horrible experiences of denial. We hate to go on diets. And if we don't lose lots of weight real quick, then our enthusiasm dies, and so does the New Year's resolution.

But remember, this isn't a diet. So why should you immediately see results? The results will come, if you want them to, and you commit yourself to the effort. So don't give up on yourself. Keep your commitment to improved health. The results will come. And once they do, once the ball gets rolling, once you begin to see the pounds disappear, your success will then be your motivation. The enthusiasm to continue an effort is easy when you can see and feel the results of your efforts. It is at the start that you must work at maintaining the effort. So, hang in there. It can work for you, IF YOU WANT IT BAD ENOUGH!

Do you now believe that the proper attitude is critical to the success of your efforts? There are some that will tell you that dieting is more an issue of what's between your ears and not so much what passes over your lips. And they're right. Attitude is critical. You have to believe in yourself. You have to want to improve your lifestyle. And that will improve the way you look. But don't kid yourself. Though attitude is important (very important in the early days of this journey), what passes over your lips is also important. The importance of the food type and quantity is something that you have to learn about and decide for yourself.

Now although I have already stated the following, I am going to repeat it because it is so very important. Remember I said it will take time to start seeing the pounds disappear. And that may be hard to handle. If you have been working at this technique for a whole week and you're seeing no results you might get discouraged. Just remember this technique is a slow process where you make very small changes in lifestyle and that is why it may take some time to see the pounds disappear. It is the slow approach that makes it much easier. It is the small changes in lifestyle that make the journey so much more enjoyable. And hopefully your good attitude will keep you working at making small changes to bring about the weight loss. In order to lose a lot of weight really fast, you have to make drastic, and probably not enjoyable, changes in your diet and lifestyle. And with this fast technique you are not developing a new lifestyle that you can continue for the rest of your life. You're dieting in the old conventional way.

Chapter 2

COMMITMENT

There's a somewhat confusing relationship between commitment and attitude. They're almost the same thing. But really they're not. More importantly, they are both equally important and absolutely necessary. That's why these two chapters are at the very beginning of the book; one right behind the other. It becomes a question of whether a person can have the right attitude without commitment. Or, stated another way, can a person have the commitment and not have the right attitude? I think you will find that both are necessary. And I believe you will find one drives the other. But you must admit that if the attitude is poor, it's probably due to a lack of commitment. Think for a moment about the two ballplayers in the previous chapter. Did they each have the right attitude and commitment? Were they each committed to getting a hit? And did that commitment, or lack of commitment, determine their attitude as they walked to the plate? Commitment and attitude are like a high performance engine and a high octane fuel. They are both required. One is not of much good without the other. The engine's performance is definitely dependent on the quality of the fuel. The stronger the commitment, the better the attitude will be. The real question is what does it take to form that all important commitment? And how much are you committed to the effort? Or, better said, how strong is your commitment?

To understand this relationship, let's examine two people. First, we have Ted who weighs about 249 pounds, is 5' 9" tall and is 32 years old. Second we have his very good friend Mike who weighs in at 320 pounds, is 6'3" tall and is 28 years old. Though Ted is a bit more "overweight" than Mike, they both need to lose a few pounds and they both know it. They kid each other about it, they talk about it, and both have probably tried various dieting techniques and exercise routines. Oops, there's that nasty word, exercise. Oh, I hate that word.

The question is if they both know they are overweight why haven't they done something about it? Let's assume they have gone to the gym together and "worked out." So why have their previous exercise routines and diets failed them in addressing this problem? And you could ask yourself this same question. If I can assume you are reading this book because you are overweight, then might you ask yourself the same question? Why, am I reading this book today? Why did I not go on a diet and lose the weight last year or the year before? What is keeping me from addressing this and losing the weight I want to lose?

What are Ted and Mike's attitudes? They both know they're too heavy. They kid each other about it. So their attitude is one of joking about the problem. They don't take their being overweight very seriously. So they're not committed to losing any weight. That's not surprising. Most of us know we are overweight. We wish we weren't. We wish we could do something about it. But for some reason we haven't done anything about it (yet). Sometimes we joke about it. Sometimes we hide behind that humor. In essence, commitment drives the attitude. You have to first make a commitment and that develops or results in your attitude. The attitude is what moves us toward achieving the goal we've committed to.

If we know we are overweight, and we dwell on that, then our attitude becomes one of concentrating on being overweight. The attitude "well I'm overweight and I'll always be overweight" rules out any chance of changing. Why? Because your concentrating on the fact that you're overweight. If you spend all of your time concentrating on your being too heavy, you will stay heavy. If the one ballplayer goes to the plate concentrating on striking out, he will probably strike out. And if this attitude stays with him no matter who is pitching, he will probably soon find he is off the team. The overweight person, like the ballplayer, definitely has an attitude. But it is an attitude about what's wrong. Or you might say they have a negative attitude. So now, we have two types of attitude. There is a negative attitude that results in our concentrating on what's wrong and therefore keeps us from progressing in the direction we really want to go. And there is a positive attitude that we develop while we are actually traveling toward the desired end (our commitment). And some, who are overweight and know it, don't have an attitude. They just accept who they are and how they look. Or, I guess you could say they have an attitude of acceptance, and that's fine. But the thing in common between the over weight person whose attitude is one of acceptance and the ballplayer's attitude of acceptance toward striking out is that neither has made a commitment to change.

Ok. So now we have determined there are three attitudes. There's the positive attitude of "I'm going to lose weight." And there's the attitude of, "I'll never be able to lose weight." And there are those who accept themselves and don't worry about it at all. It's not that they don't care. They really do care. They're just not concerned about their overweight condition. They accept themselves as they are and that's fine. And if that's the case, they're probably not reading this book. But you are reading this book. So, let's assume your attitude is not one of acceptance.

What about commitment? Are there different commitments? Is there a negative commitment, a lack of commitment, as well as a positive commitment? I seriously doubt it. I don't believe anyone is committed to being overweight. It may seem that way to an outsider, since they don't see the person doing anything about it. But if you were to ask, most people will tell you they would love to be slimmer. There not necessarily unhappy with themselves or the way they look. Many people are very happy with who they are and how they look. But even those who are happy with themselves and their appearance will admit that for no other reason than health, it would be best is they were a few pounds lighter. If you were able to wave a magic wand over their head and "poof" they would instantly lose weight, I doubt if they would ask you to not perform your magic over them. So, as far as commitment goes, you are either committed to something or you're not.

Okay. So now it's a question of changing our attitude, and making a commitment. Or making a commitment first and having that result in the drive to succeed (our positive attitude). Gee that was easy. But how do we change our attitude? And how do we make a commitment? Or better said, what causes us to make a commitment. If you ask someone who was overweight and has slimmed down, how they did it. They will tell you all about the diet; what they ate; how much they ate; what pills they took; what exercises they performed at the gym, and on and on. But what they will not tell you is what took place that made them decide (the commitment) to lose weight. What was the event that triggered the process and made them commit, all of a sudden, to losing weight? They, like most people, were probably overweight for some time. Why didn't they lose the weight a year before, or two years before? What happened to them that all of a sudden they made a commitment to lose weight? How did that mental change take place? What caused it? Why did they all of a sudden stop devoting their attention to being overweight and devote their attention to losing weight?

If you were to talk to Ted and Mike a year later and found that Ted now weighs 165 pounds and Mike now weighs 275, you would want to know how they did it. You want to know something? How they did it is not as important as <u>why</u> they did it. What caused them to stop concentrating on being overweight and concentrate on losing the weight?   You will find that every single person who at one time was overweight and has lost that weight had an incident or some special occurrence that made them address the problem.

Something happened that caused the commitment. It was "the trigger" that caused Ted to address his obesity. And I believe it's important for you to determine precisely what has made you, or hopefully will, make you (in the future), address your issue. Why are you reading this?

In Ted's case, he may have overheard one of his son's friends talking about how fat his dad is. It's okay for Ted to kid himself about his obesity. And Mike and Ted can kid each other about it. But to hear someone else say it, hurts. And when Ted heard that conversation between his son and his son's friend, he decided to do something about it. That was the birth of his commitment. But if his attitude is still one of concentrating on being overweight, his commitment will not carry him very far into the journey. He must start thinking about being thin. He must develop an attitude of hitting the home run. If he concentrates on striking out, he surely will. So Ted started concentrating on those positive things he was doing; eating better, including fewer beers with Mike; getting active. He started thinking about where he wanted to be rather than were he was right now. His attention was on the new Ted and not the old Ted. No more thoughts of Ted the fat guy. He was Ted the thin guy. It is the attitude that will carry him forward. And the attitude was formed by his new commitment. And his commitment was triggered by the realization that he was overweight. And though he knew it for some time, hearing someone else say it drove it home.

And what about Mike's weight loss? Well Mike was jealous. He saw Ted losing the weight and he decided he would do the same. But his commitment wasn't as strong. If fact, his commitment didn't exist. He just wanted to lose weight because he saw how much better Ted was looking. He had an attitude of jealousy. But he was not committed to losing weight. He lost a few pounds, but wasn't really "into it," if you know what I mean. At least that was the case until he hurt his knee and during treatment of that injury, the doctor found a problem with his heart. At that moment, Ted also made a commitment. And in the next 26 weeks, he shed 45 pounds.

Another possibility, and this is quite common between guys, is that they both lost the weight because they bet each other that they could lose more weight. And often this works. Parents may challenge their children to lose weight by promising a reward. Companies often issue rewards to employees who improve their health through losing weight. Here, the company benefits in reduced healthcare costs. The only problem is that the commitment is more based on financial elements than on improved health. And if Ted and Mike lost the weight because their company rewarded them with $100, what are they chances that they truly realize the weight loss is critical to their health. What's important to them is the hundred bucks in their wallet. Health wasn't the real reason they lost the weight, so their improved health will probably not be much of an incentive to keep the weight off. The goal was $100.00, not improved health.

Though Ted and Mike are fictitious characters, there journey is identical to that of many others who have successfully lost weight. I tell their story to drive home the following points. Most everyone who is overweight has been that way for some time. The fact that you have not been able to do something about it is very natural. Maybe you're not ready yet. Maybe the commitment is just not there (yet). If you think I'm describing you, then read to the end of this chapter and stop. And don't come back to read the next chapters for at least two days.

During those days stop thinking of yourself as someone who is overweight. If you think all the time about being overweight, you're concentrating on what's wrong. You're thinking about striking out. For the next two days think of yourself as Ted. Think only about who you would like to become. Concentrate only on that. Picture yourself as a thin you. Think about all the new and beautiful clothes you will need. Think about how people will notice the new you and compliment you. Stop thinking about what you see in the mirror today. Think of looking in that mirror on some future day and being pleased with what you see.

But do one thing. Weigh yourself right now and record the weight right here. As you will see, it is important to know and record your weight right now. My weight on (today's date) _____________ is _____________pounds. Remember, for the next couple of days think only of who you want to become and not of who you are.

In essence, I'm asking you to think, over the next two days, about making a commitment. We've all heard the old joke about which came first, the chicken or the egg? Well the same can be asked about commitment and attitude. Which comes first? Well, here's the defining statement about commitment and attitude. Commitment comes first. Your attitude toward losing weight, the chances of success in taking this journey, is one-hundred percent totally dependent on the strength of your commitment to succeed. And if, after two days, you still can't make a commitment, then put this book on a shelf and forget about it. You're just not ready … yet.

Chapter 3

MY JOURNEY

I'm going to take some time now and describe my journey, and how this process of lifestyle change came about for me. It's important to understand why I committed myself to losing weight and how I discovered the processes and techniques that I will ask you to undertake.

This process started for me in the late fall of 1974. That's when I went to my doctor and he discovered my blood pressure was practically off the scale. It wasn't much of a surprise to me since I had received the same warning from doctors in years previous. But when he stated that I didn't have much of a chance of living another five or six years, it got to me. I began to relate his comment to my general health. The fact that I was always tired and having difficulties playing with my children didn't faze me at the time. And the fact that going up a flight of stairs took my breath didn't seem all that unusual. But then I began to relate these issues to the doctor's warning. These were issues I had noticed. At the time they didn't they seem life threatening. But now, it was a different story.

I had tried every diet you can think of, including hypnosis. I lost weight on some of them. But I could never keep the weight off. Why? Well I think it's because as soon as the diet was over, I went right back to the original life-style that resulted in my being overweight. And believe me I have some of the most horrible eating habits in the world. I don't like, nor will I eat, salads. Everything I love is fattening. I don't like most of the things that are good for me. And, if it isn't fried, I probably won't like it, and I guarantee, I will not eat it. So, I was, in the long run, unsuccessful in losing weight. I just never learned to change my eating habits for a healthier life.

Knowing this, I asked my doctor for some help. He prescribed an appetite suppressant for me. But, he said that he would only give it to me for a limited time to get me started. Beyond that point he said I had to do it myself. He knew that I could not live the rest of my life on appetite suppressants. So, with the help of those pills I began eating less food. Since I wasn't going to stop eating the things I loved, I had to eat less. To a small degree I began watching what I was eating as well. But all of those healthy things that dieters are supposed to eat were not going to get near my mouth. I don't like them. I will never like them. And therefore, I will not eat them. So I had to just eat less. And the appetite suppressant helped in achieving that.

Over the next several months I did lose weight going from somewhere around 250 pounds down to 230 pounds. I don't remember my actual weight when I started this traditional "diet," because I had avoided the scale. In fact, I had been avoiding the scale for years. Why? I knew I was overweight. I didn't need a scale to tell me I was too fat. I saw it every time I looked in a mirror. What was a scale going to tell me that I didn't already know? I was just never at that point where I was ready to do something about it; until now. But I do know that I weighed very close to, if not over, 250 pounds. And for a man who is 5'10' tall, that's a dangerous weight. I was roughly 75 pounds overweight.

I also took up golf. GOLF? That isn't exercise! You're right it isn't a very physical activity. Nowhere near as strenuous as jogging or cycling or aerobics. Given my condition, jogging or aerobics would have probably killed me. So I took up golf and I walked the golf course. I refused to ride in a golf cart. Okay. Sometimes I had to ride, because of the crowded conditions on the golf course and because at certain times, the course rules will not permit you to walk. It is just too slow. But most courses will let you walk the course in the early evening. So, I began getting just this little bit of activity a couple of evenings a week, and started losing weight. I wasn't able to undertake more strenuous activities since I had undergone spinal surgery a few years prior.   As a side note, I also learned over the following months that my weight was a major contributor to my continuing back problems.

I did try to reduce the amount of candy bars, doughnuts, ice cream, and things of that nature. But at mealtime, I did not change my eating habits other than eating less. And eating less was something the pills helped me realize. Later on, I began changing my eating habits to a larger degree, but not at this early stage. I had several lessons to learn first. But we'll get to that later. But I had definitely taught myself to eat smaller quantities.

So, with the help of the appetite suppressant I was losing weight and I was very pleased with my progress. But I was also finding that the medication was having adverse effects. So I decided to stop taking the pills and hoped that I could continue to lose weight at the same rate I had been losing. The key to this whole process is in that last statement. And the key is the word <u>rate</u>.

What exactly is rate? Rate is the measurement of something per some unit of time. For example, if you lose two and one-half pounds in a single week, then your weight loss is two and one-half pounds lost <u>per</u> week.   I underlined the word "per" because that defines the measurement over time. Most people indicate rates by using a graph. So, I decided to make a graph, with weight on the vertical axis, and the days of the month on the horizontal axis. Here's a typical graph for a 30 day period.

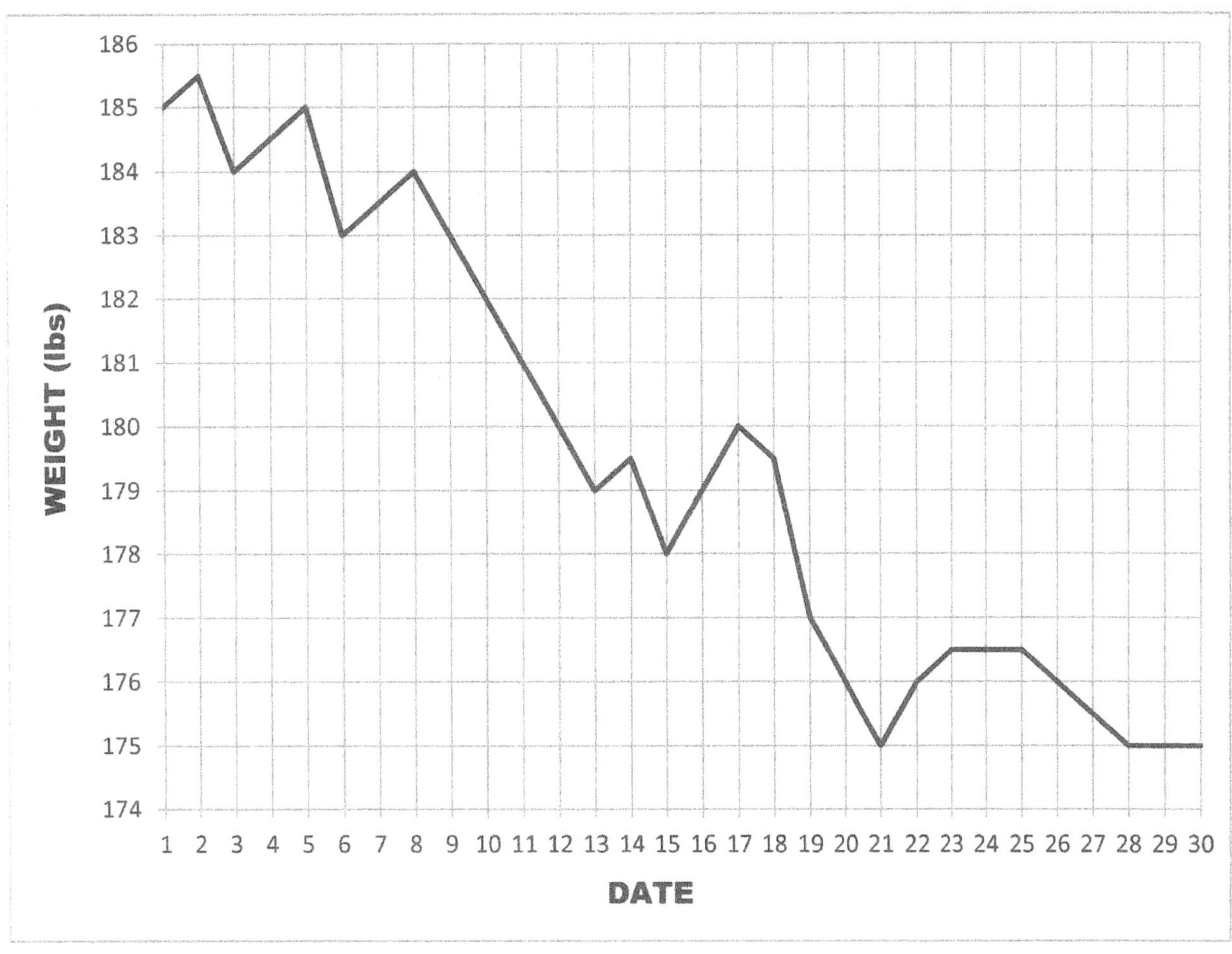

The graph is a good indicator of the amount of weight lost, and the period of time it has taken to lose that weight. That is the rate. So, I started thinking, "I wonder if I can control the rate at which I lose weight?" It was around Christmas and I had lost 20 pounds over the three previous months. So I decided on January 1st I would stop taking the appetite suppressants and try to continue losing weight. Now I had lost about 20 pounds over three months. That means I was losing weight at a rate of six and two thirds (6 2/3) pounds per month. The rate is calculated by dividing 20 (pounds) by 3 (months). So I began to figure "let's see, if I lose about ten pounds a month, then by summer (6 months) I could lose another 60 pounds." And the only way I could think of looking at these figures and to see how my weight loss was going, in comparison to this goal, was to draw a graph, and plot my daily weight. And that was the birth of my weight graph.

Though I had avoided the scale, it was obvious that I was going to have to weigh myself quite often to ensure that I was continuing to lose weight at the rate I wanted. Many diets tell you not to weigh yourself every day. The reason for this is simple. They don't want you to lose your enthusiasm (lose your commitment and develop a negative attitude) by getting on the scale and seeing the same weight that you saw yesterday. Or maybe even see a weight that is greater than yesterday's weight. That disappointment or anger drives some people right to the refrigerator. But I had made a commitment. I was beginning to like what I saw in the mirror and I was committed to continuing this process without the pills.

I'm going to insert a warning here. I hate to break the continuity of talking about the graph, but this is extremely important and must be stated. I've talked about the danger of rapid weight loss, and will continue to do so. It is true, that by the end of December I had lost 20 pounds, and I began thinking about losing another 60 pounds over the next six months. Losing too much weight too fast is dangerous. And as you will read later, I paid a price for my rapid weight loss with a visit to the hospital.

Now before we get started plotting your graph, let's get realistic. Losing 80 pounds in nine months is expecting a lot. Even I really believed that was too much and too quick. So, common sense took over and I decided to try and continue losing about six and two-thirds pounds per month. That would put me at about 190 pounds by mid-summer. So I hoped to lose another 40 pounds, which when added to the 20 I had already lost would mean I was going to lose 60 pounds.   In my case, that would be a miracle.

I had planned a vacation in mid July and decided that I wanted to be at or below 190 pounds by July 15th. That was my **goal**. Here is a six month graph showing my "goal" weight starting on January 1st at 230 pounds and ending on July 15th at a weight of 190 pounds. In order to make the graph readable, the vertical axis has a line every five pounds and the horizontal axis has a line for every seven days. I'll call this the goal line.

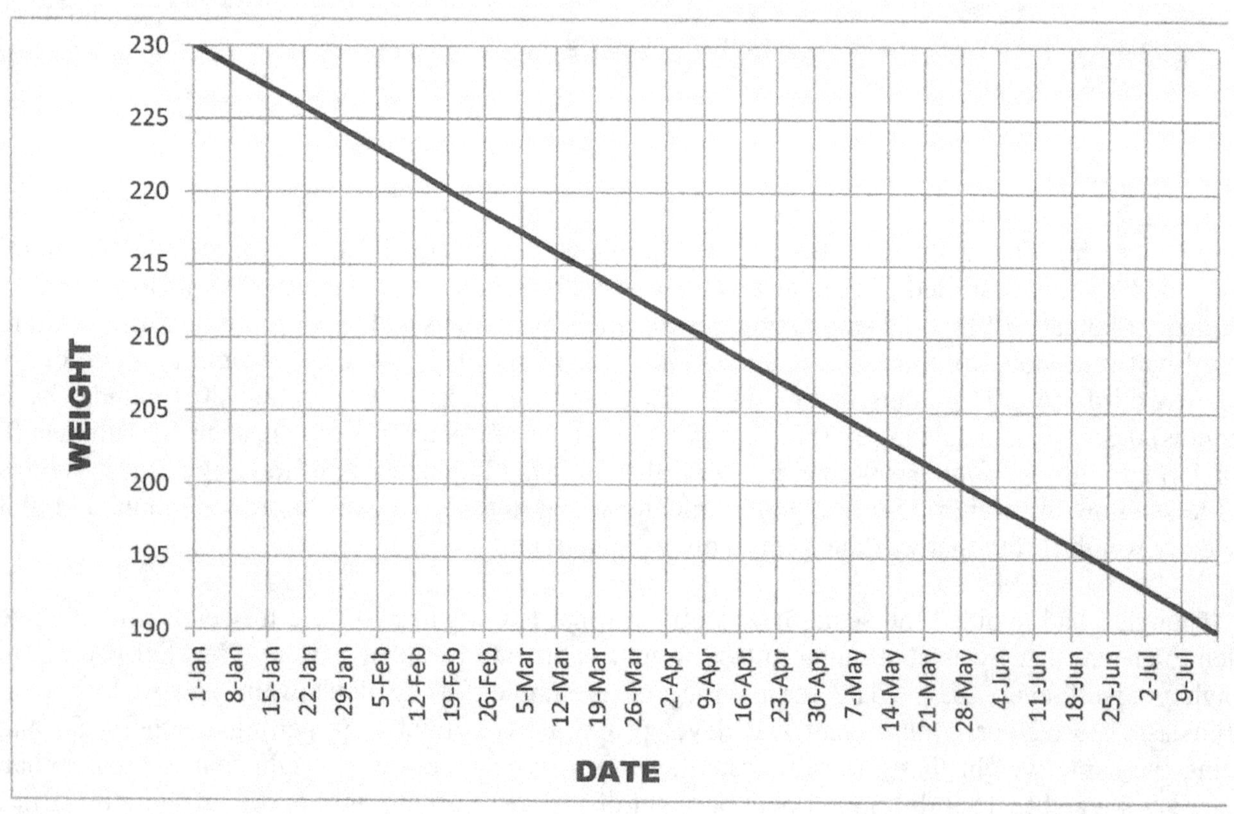

This graph is just to show you the desired rate at which I had hoped to lose weight. It is not a usable graph. It would be very difficult to record on this graph the weight taken each day. So what is really needed is a graph for each month. You will see these monthly graphs in the next chapters.

Chapter 4

THE GRAPH

Before we start making your graph, here are some thoughts about daily weighing.   It is important to measure and record your weight every day. It is in using this technique that you can begin to see the positive and negative effects that your life style has on your weight. It is absolutely necessary that you weigh yourself each and every day. To get a good feel for the way your body is affected by your living habits, I want you on the scale every morning. If you don't see any weight loss over some period, then it should, and eventually will (if you've made a solid commitment), be the driving force in making a slight change in the way you live today, so that eventually, maybe tomorrow, you will see a weight loss.

So, to get started, get a piece of graph paper. You can buy this type of paper at all kinds of stores from variety stores to drug stores. They have it in the school supply department. And I would not advise getting the kind of paper that is labeled "graph paper." What I would look for is a tablet of paper that has blue lines (both vertical and horizontal) printed on the page. The blue lines are about a quarter on an inch apart and cover the entire 8 ½ X 11 inch sheet.

As I describe this, look at the opposing page to see two of my graphs. On the left side of the paper draw a vertical line about an inch in from the edge. At the very top, just to the left of the vertical line you have drawn, record your present weight plus two pounds. Then on the next line down, write your weight plus one pound. On the next line down, record your present weight. Continue this on down the left edge to the bottom of the page reducing the number by one pound.

Across the bottom of the page, draw a horizontal line about an inch up from the bottom edge. Here you will write the days of the month. Starting at the extreme left, right below the vertical line you made, write today's date. At the bottom of the next printed vertical line, write tomorrows date. Continue this across the entire page. This is your weight graph. You can make one for each month, or you could, if your paper is large enough, make one for several months. I taped several pieces of graph paper together and made a graph for six months. On the opposing page are my two graphs for January and February. They show the actual weight measured each day and the goal weight (goal line). The challenge is to stay below that goal line. And this is where the discoveries lie. You will begin to determine and learn what it takes to stay below your goal line. This is where you will educate yourself and begin to formulate a new lifestyle to ensure you don't go above your goal line.

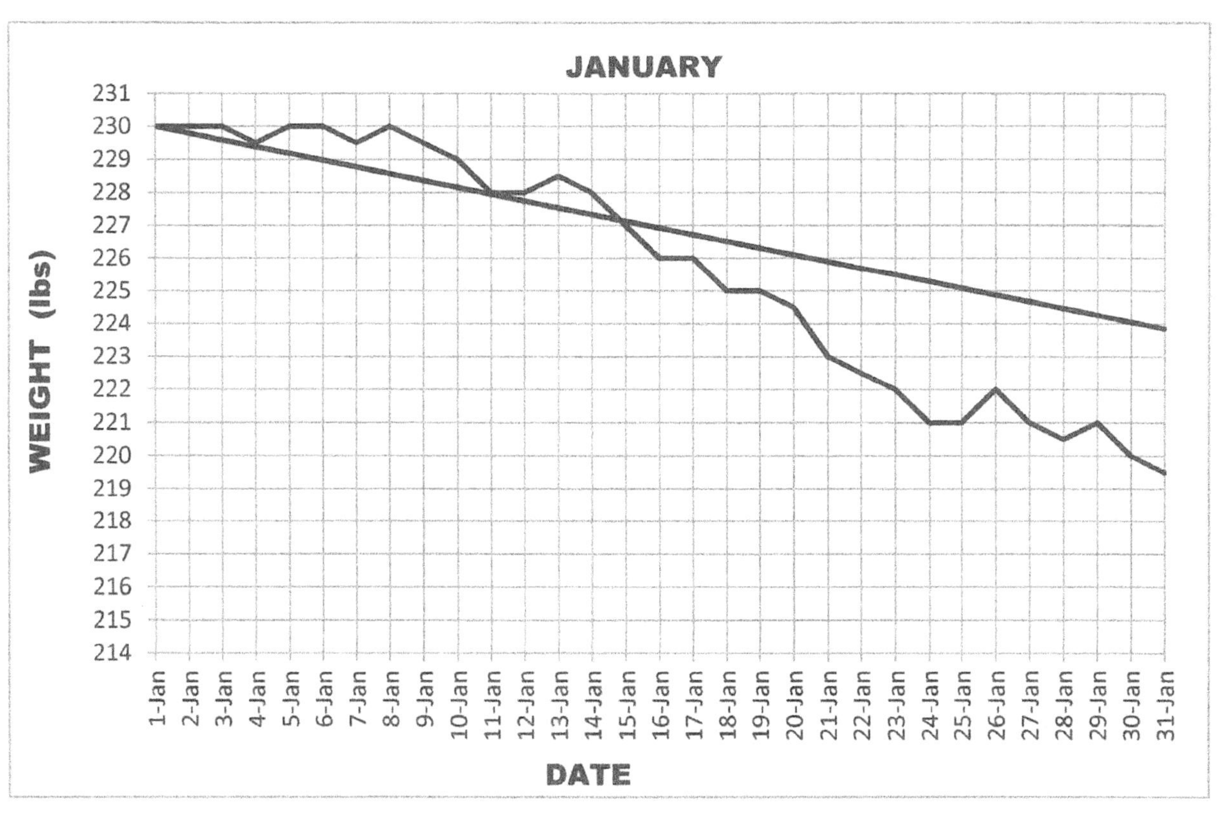
JANUARY
WEIGHT (lbs)
231
230
229
228
227
226
225
224
223
222
221
220
219
218
217
216
215
214
1-Jan
2-Jan
3-Jan
4-Jan
5-Jan
6-Jan
7-Jan
8-Jan
9-Jan
10-Jan
11-Jan
12-Jan
13-Jan
14-Jan
15-Jan
16-Jan
17-Jan
18-Jan
19-Jan
20-Jan
21-Jan
22-Jan
23-Jan
24-Jan
25-Jan
26-Jan
27-Jan
28-Jan
29-Jan
30-Jan
31-Jan
DATE

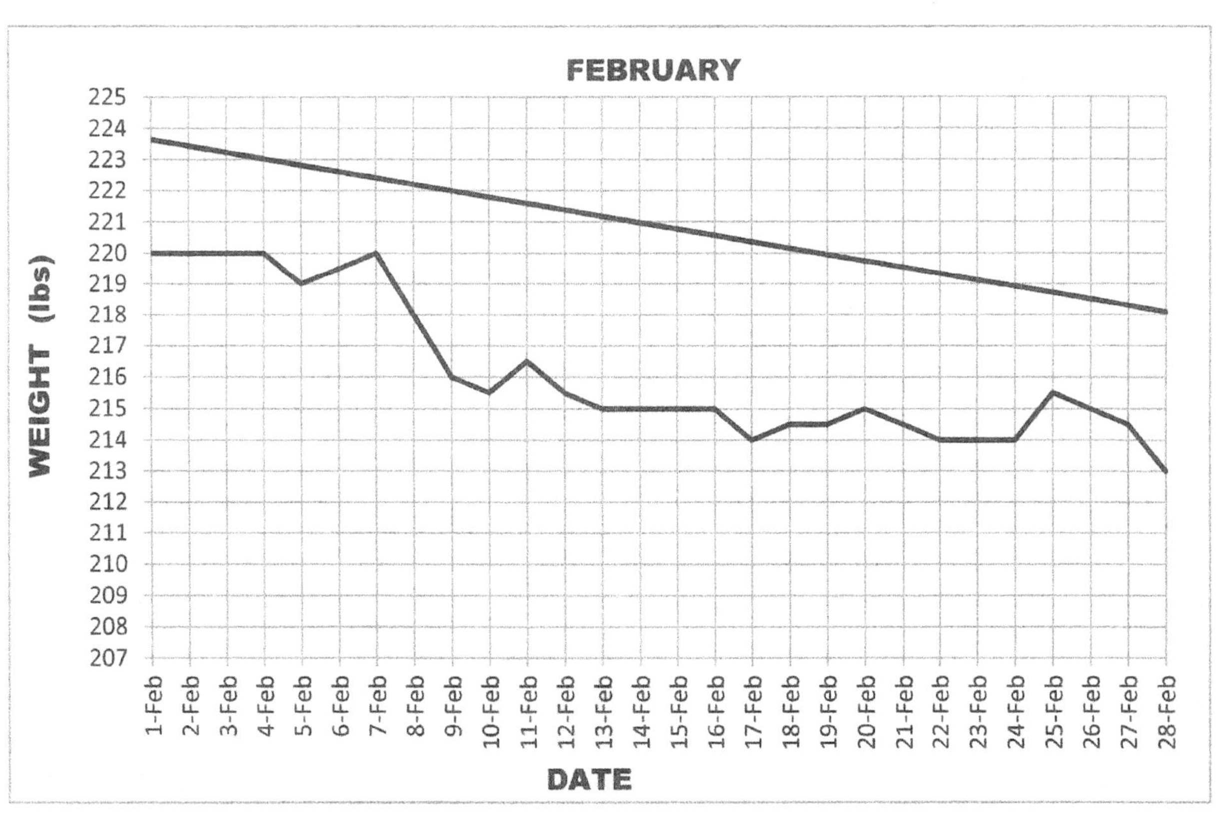
FEBRUARY
WEIGHT (lbs)
225
224
223
222
221
220
219
218
217
216
215
214
213
212
211
210
209
208
207
1-Feb
2-Feb
3-Feb
4-Feb
5-Feb
6-Feb
7-Feb
8-Feb
9-Feb
10-Feb
11-Feb
12-Feb
13-Feb
14-Feb
15-Feb
16-Feb
17-Feb
18-Feb
19-Feb
20-Feb
21-Feb
22-Feb
23-Feb
24-Feb
25-Feb
26-Feb
27-Feb
28-Feb
DATE

John Borntraeger

Chapter 5

THE ENVELOPE

As you can see from the graphs for January and February, I was losing weight at a rate greater than the six and two-thirds pounds a month I was shooting for. I asked myself, "why not shoot for something a little better?" I hadn't seen 180 pounds since my high school days, except to see the number go "whizzing" by when I got on the scale. But I wanted to get down to 178 pounds, since that was the weight my doctor had said was the upper recommended weight for a person my age and height. Let's see 230 pounds to 178 pounds . . . that's 52 pounds over six and one-half months or, about eight and two-third pounds per month. And figuring there are 196 days in those six and one-half months, that's about 0.25 (one-quarter) pounds per day. That seems a little excessive. But I thought to myself, "What the heck." "It's a goal." "It's something to shoot for." So, I found the 178 pound point on my graph on July 15th. From that point I drew a line to my weight of 230 pounds on January 1st. Then I found the 190 pound point on July 15th (my first goal) and drew a second line from that point to the weight of 230 pounds on January 1st. Here's the graph for six months showing the envelope made up of the two goal lines.

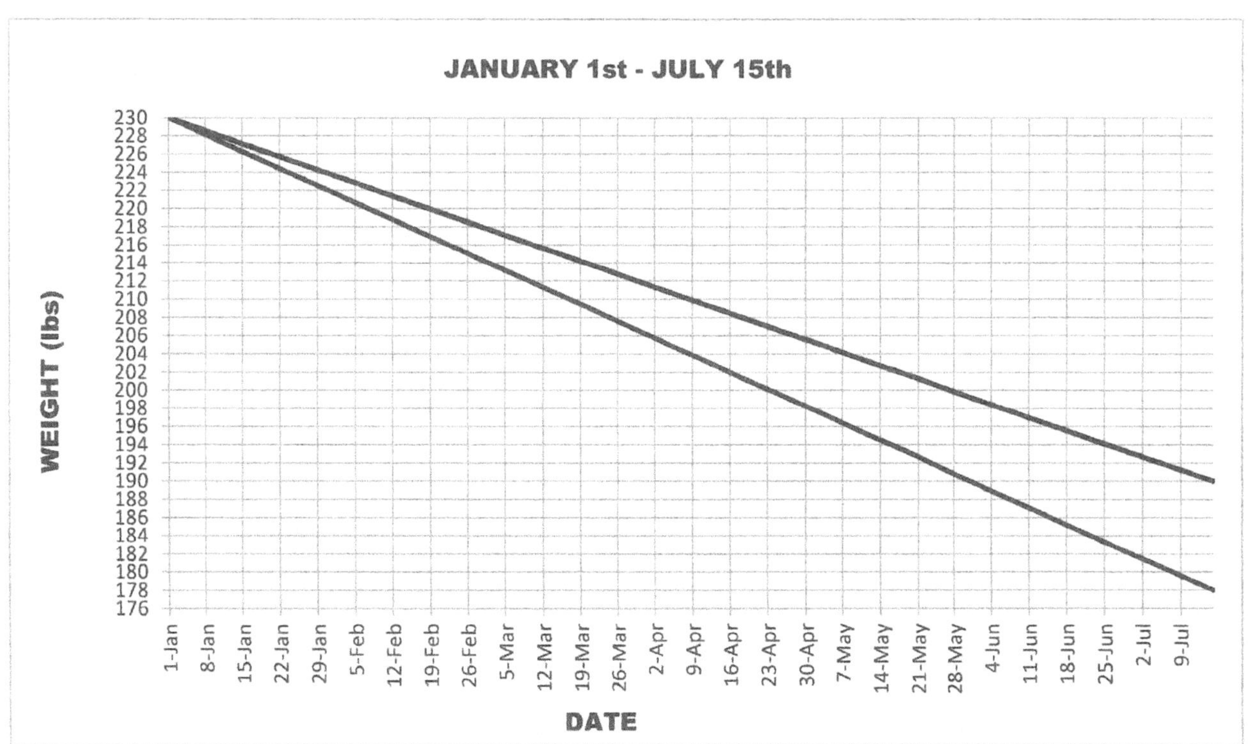

This graph shows the two slopping lines both starting at 230 pounds. One stops at 190, the second stops at 178. What I suggest, is that you draw these two lines in RED on your graph.

This became my envelope. It became my goal to keep my weight always inside those two goal lines. If I could do that, my diet would be a success. Notice that at this point, I was still thinking of this experience as a diet. Why? Well, I, like most people, had been taught to think that way. I was going to try and lose some weight. That, by definition, is a diet. It wasn't until much later that I began thinking about my experiences, changes in eating habits and activity habits, and realized that I had not been on a diet, as we know it

I will discuss throughout this book the many things I learned from this experience. It is all these things that made me realize that starting January 1st, I wasn't on a diet. I can say this because those things that constitute a diet, as we know it, were the least important things during my experience. They had to be! I wasn't about to eat all those things that were "good for me." If I don't like it, I'm not going to eat it. And I wasn't going to give up all the things I love. Yet, I did lose weight. Therefore, I say my experience was not a diet (as we know it).

Well, for now, let's get back to the pair of goal lines, the envelope. That envelope was the basis for the beginning of my education in living habits. As I monitored my daily weight, I began to learn what it took to stay inside those two goal lines; what various things I might do to lose control and go above the top goal line; and many techniques for maintaining the rate at which I wanted to lose weight. Here are my weight graphs for January and February with the envelope added.

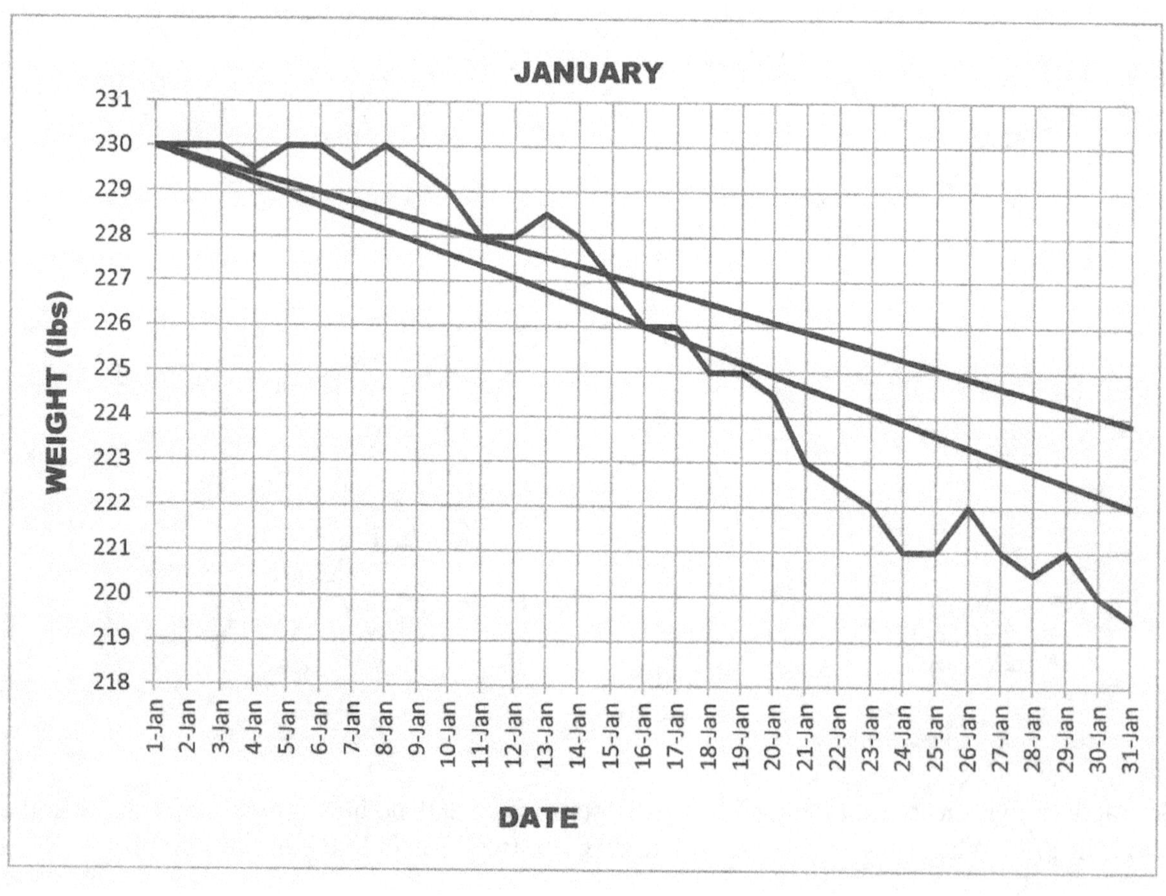

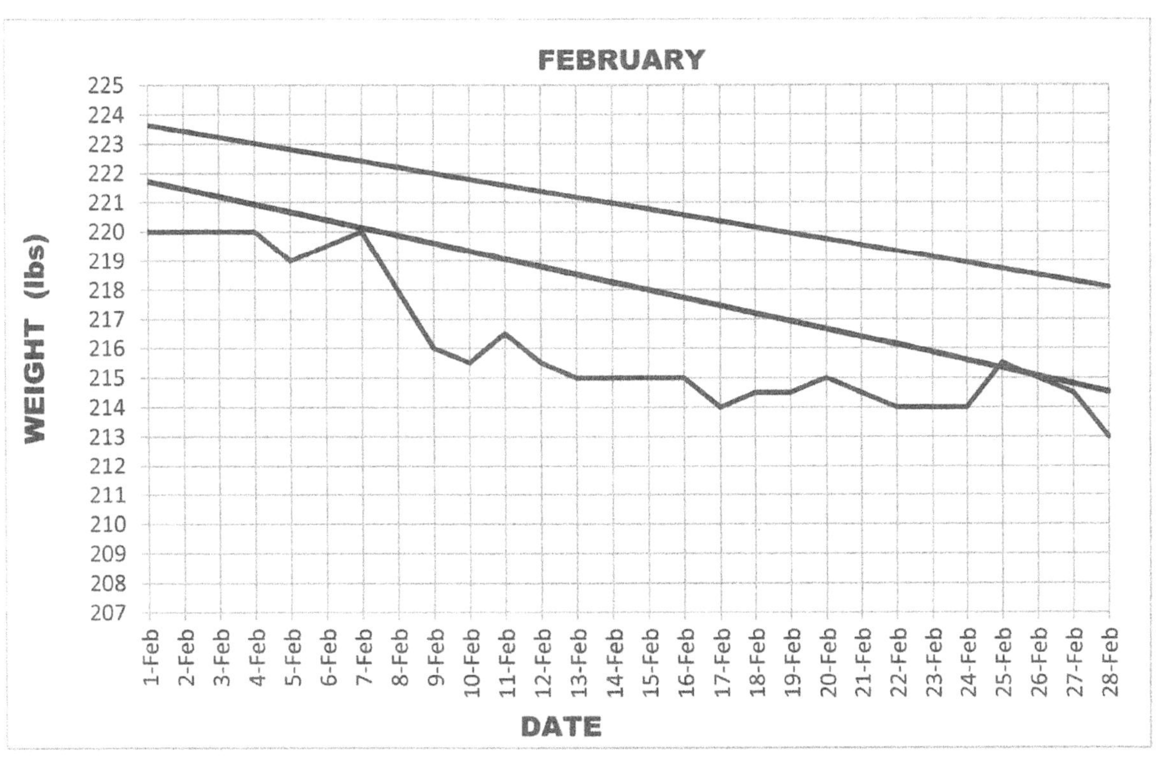

You will notice that the two slopping lines definitely define the rate at which I planned to lose excess pounds. Remember, you must challenge yourself, but not so much that you lessen your chances of success. For if you over-challenge yourself, you'll get discouraged. And that discouragement can negatively affect your commitment and result in an attitude of, "I just can't lose weight!" Remember, the upper line of your envelope is your goal. The lower line represents nothing more than an even greater challenge. You will also learn that the lower line serves as a maximum loss rate. Losing weight at a greater rate (going below the lower goal line) can be detrimental to your health. So, think of going above the top goal line as dangerous to the success of your efforts and going below the lower goal line as DANGEROUS to your health. And I mean this in all sincerity!

Constantly working to stay inside those two goal lines is the key to this whole process. You MUST teach yourself what is necessary to stay inside your envelope. You must also seriously analyze what factors (eating habits and activity habits) contribute to your going above the top goal line. But, since we have agreed this must be done slowly, it is NOT difficult to do this.

But you must make a COMMITMENT and you must maintain a "can do" ATTITUDE.

Chapter 6

THE SLOWDOWN

If you looked real closely at the graphs for January and February, you may have noticed a drop in the rate at which I was losing weight. In January I lost ten and one-half pounds and in February I lost only seven pounds. And in March it got even worse. In March I lost only three pounds going from 213 on the 1st to 210 pounds on the 31st.

This is quite common. And, it is where you have to learn to take control. Most people tend to lose more weight in the early stages. There are probably a number of reasons for this. One of course, is the enthusiasm and excitement of the success that sort of carries you along for a while. Then, we get somewhat complacent. You almost think that this whole process is automatic. Once you start losing weight, it will just magically continue to disappear. But it doesn't. You have to make additional changes to ensure you continue to lose weight.

I also thought that maybe I had over-challenged myself. I mentioned in a previous chapter that over-challenging can lead to failure. If you try to lose weight at a rate that is faster than your capable of losing, then you risk losing the proper attitude and just quitting.

In looking at my graph for March, it becomes quite evident that I had gotten complacent and was not losing weight. From March 10th through March 24th (a period of over two weeks) I was unable to lose any additional weight.

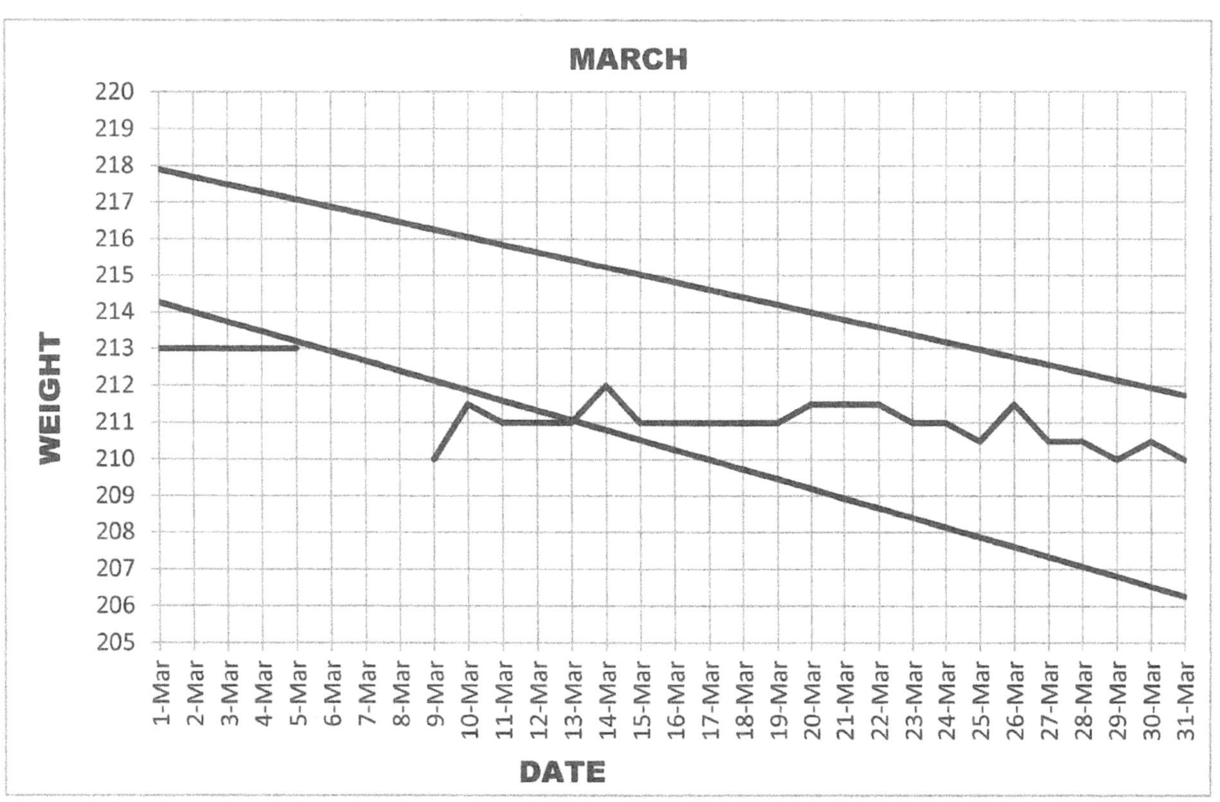

You may also note that on March 6th, 7th and 8th there is no weight entered on the chart. Well, that's because I was in the hospital suffering from kidney stones. So, though I was upset about not continuing to lose weight in March at the rate I had achieved in January and February, it's quite possible that the weight loss rate in March was a lot better for my total health than that of January and February.

It was in late March during a visit with my doctor, concerning the kidney stone episode, that the relationship between my weight loss and the kidney stone attack was discussed. His recommendation that I drink at least eight glasses of water a day was followed from that point on. I'll talk a bit more about this episode in the hospital in a later chapter.

At this same time I realized that I had to do more to increase the rate at which I was losing weight. In January and February I was able to stay (except for one day) below the lower goal line. But in March I entered the envelope and toward the end of March I noticed that I was moving closer to the upper goal line. And I did not want to go above my envelope. So, toward the end of March I began to stop eating some of the items that I believed were keeping me from continuing to lose weight. In addition, spring had begun and I was able to start walking the golf course a bit more often.

It is these little decisions that you will make that determine the success and make it so easy to follow this process. As you see yourself approaching the upper goal line, you decide to eat fewer desserts, or stop them altogether. It is your decision to add some additional activity, or stop eating bread or french fries, or whatever. It is the intelligent choices about your lifestyle that makes the system work and makes it an enjoyable journey. And, again, it all has to do with commitment and attitude.

Chapter 7

THE EFFORT

As I stated earlier, no one can lose weight or change his or her living habits without making an effort. The degree of effort you make is totally dependent upon your mental attitude and your commitment. Changing your living habits can be done in very small degrees, with equally small results. There is nothing wrong with this approach. It may very well be the key to your success, in that it makes this experience pleasant. The danger of making major changes is that the experience becomes unpleasant, unhealthy, and has little chance of success.

If you went so far as to say to yourself: "Okay. From now on, no bread, ice cream, soda, potatoes, candy, beer, butter or margarine, pastries, peanut butter, and anything fried" you would be miserable. I know I would. If I stopped eating the above items, I would die since I also am not going to eat the things I don't like. For me, there would be nothing left. You don't have to give up the things you like. All you have to do is learn to eat these things in moderation. At least that's the best way to get started. Just try and reduce the quantity of those things that you know are fattening. You may even stop eating these things altogether once you start seeing the pounds disappear and begin to feel better about yourself. I did stop eating some things. Others I love and will never stop eating. But I have learned to eat them in moderation, because I know the consequences if I eat too much of these things.

So, to start your effort, try reducing the amounts of these types of things and also increase your daily activity. At lunch time, take just twenty minutes and walk. I found that after just two weeks, I could walk 15 blocks in twenty to thirty minutes. You have no idea the number of calories you burn with a brisk twenty minute walk. You also have no idea how a frequent but short walk can help to flatten your stomach.

This experience, be it successful or unsuccessful, depends totally upon your effort (commitment and attitude). I'm afraid it's not what you hoped for. I don't know of any way to shed pounds without making an effort. There is no technique of going to sleep and waking up 50 pounds lighter; no magic wand. Although, and we'll talk about this a little later, sleep can be a positive factor in losing weight.

So, start by increasing your physical activity. Nothing strenuous; just do a little more. Take a walk, or take a bike ride. And also, instead of having two doughnuts with your morning coffee, have just one. With your eggs, have whole wheat toast, and put a little less butter on it.

If you do this, you'll discover something. First, the increased physical activity will make you feel better. And second, you won't want that second doughnut. Why? Well, two reasons come to mind. The first reason is that you realize, "if I eat that second doughnut, then the twenty minute walk I took yesterday is wasted. Why would I take that walk only to destroy my effort with this doughnut?" The second reason is also the second discovery. You feel good about yourself. You feel good about your effort. It is that good feeling about yourself that helps keep you going. What's another word for that "good feeling?" It's attitude. And when you see the pounds begin to disappear, you will then really feel good about yourself. And the better you feel, the more you'll do to change the way you look and the way you live. Does the following statement sound familiar? The commitment gets you started. An ever increasingly good attitude keeps you going.

This then becomes like the snow ball rolling down the hill. It starts as a tiny flake of snow blowing in the wind. As it rolls along the ground it gets bigger then begins rolling down a hill. As it rolls down the hill, it picks up more snow and gets bigger. As it gets bigger, it also gets heavier and rolls faster and faster, picking up more snow and getting bigger and so on and so on. The changes in your living habits and the way you look and feel both physically and mentally (about yourself and your effort) begin to have a positive effect on each other. They stimulate each other and they fuel each other. Much like the snowball, as you begin to see results of your efforts, your efforts become easier, and you will tend to do more for your well-being. Reducing the amount of certain food types won't be an unpleasant chore, it will become something you want to do. When this type of decision becomes easy, you have shifted your mental attitude from denial to intelligent choices. You will have begun the task of changing your living habits. And because your efforts are undertaken slowly and in small incremental steps, it is a lifestyle that you can and will continue forever. So again, you will realize there is no end to this process. There are ends to "diets." But since you are not on a diet and are changing the way you live, there is no end to this process. Once you lose weight and feel fantastic about yourself and your appearance, why would you want it to end?

Okay. Let's talk about the activity side of this lifestyle change. It seems strange, but the same thing happens to people who begin new physical activities. They seem to undergo the same type of change in mental attitudes. I remember hearing an interview with a fellow who was probably the first true "jogger." This was before the jogging craze hit this country. He stated that when he was out running, he felt so much better about everything. It improved his mental attitude about everything. He stated that when he was running, he felt almost euphoric. People who have been on drugs talk about a "high" they experience when on the drugs. Runners talk about this same type of "high." In fact, the medical profession is finding that people who suffer from depression undergo positive changes in their mental state when they exercise. Scientific evidence has been discovered that there are certain chemicals released in the brain or released elsewhere in the body and sent to the brain that positively affect mental attitude. So, it is true that physical activity can and does have a positive affect on us physically and mentally. But remember, and I can't emphasize this enough, you should see your doctor before making any major changes in your physical activity.

What's a major change? That depends on you. A minor change for someone 28 years old could be a major undertaking for someone who is 60 years old. Consult your physician. He or she knows best what you are capable of doing at the outset. And, be careful. Don't overdo this physical activity thing. You're not trying to kill yourself. You're trying to gradually change your lifestyle. Do it in small increments. That way you have a much better chance of continuing this particular lifestyle modification for years to come. And I have another bonus for you. If you take a short walk, there will come a time that you will look forward to your walk, and will be saddened if it's raining and you can't take that walk. I know. I've experienced it. If you had told me before I started this journey that I would be saddened by not being able to take a walk I would have told you that you were totally nuts.

So, it does take effort and it does take commitment. Oops, there's that word again. But somewhere along the road, it will no longer be an effort. That's when attitude takes over. Oops, there's that other word again. And when this happens, you will have successfully started changing your life-style. And how will this change affect you? Brother! I could write volumes and volumes about the change in me. After having lived a life of obesity, I experienced changes that I just can't put in words. My self esteem changed, and I began to enjoy life for the first time. I could walk down a street and not worry who was looking at me. I didn't care. I felt good about me. A feeling I had never experienced. And because I had performed this miracle without going through some miserable experience, I was able to keep the pounds off. And I will always keep the pounds off. Having experienced both sides of this fence, I know which side I want to live on, and I know how to stay on the healthy side of the fence. I taught myself through this experience that I can change who I am, by slowly changing how I live.   And to my surprise, my back problems practically disappeared. My neurosurgeon put it in perspective when he said to me, "You're surprised that losing 75 pounds makes your back feel better?" "Try putting a couple of bowling balls on a chain and put the chain around your neck and see if your back doesn't start hurting." You see I had gone from a 46 inch waist to a 36 inch waist. That's a lot of weight that has to be supported by the spine. Why do you think pregnant women have such severe back aches in the later months of their pregnancy?

So, now is the time for you to decide how much effort you are willing to make. The amount of effort and the commitment you are willing to put into this effort will determine the slope of the two goal lines on your graph. I recommend that you not try and lose more than five or so pounds a month. Why? There are two reasons for the recommendation. First, slow is a better, physical choice. Rapid weight loss is unhealthy. And, second you are going to change your life-style, and that must be done slowly. Consider this. It took many years for you to develop into who you are today. Don't expect to change that overnight. You can't. You might try and change rapidly, but chances are that you will fall back into your old life-style rather quickly. So, slow going is a must. And also, the experience will be much more enjoyable. By starting slowly, your expectations will not be so high that disappointment easily sets in. And guess what. By setting your weight loss at a reasonable rate at the outset, your chances of success are much greater. And that is the key to maintaining the attitude and commitment. And if all goes well, meaning you ARE going to make that effort, you will lose weight at a rate faster than hoped for. And that's the beauty of the process. At some point in time you will find that the process is no longer driving you to lose weight. You will find that you have taken over and you dictate to the process what you want to happen. In other words, at some point in time during this journey you are about to undertake, you will be in total control of your lifestyle and bad habits will no longer control you.

There is also the danger of not setting your goal high enough. On the graph, this would be drawing your goal lines almost horizontal. If you decide to lose only a few pounds per month, you have not challenged yourself enough. You will, if you get on the scale each day and, over a period of ten days, see no weight loss; say to yourself, "that's okay. I've got next week to lose a pound. I won't worry about it now." I have news for you. You won't worry about it next week either. Why? Well, because you haven't made a commitment. And your attitude of, "I'll do better next week" is really saying, "I don't care." It's identical to the two guys in Chapter one, Ted and Mike saying to each other, "We'll start our diet next week."

Your desired weight loss rate MUST be sufficient to challenge you. You MUST make a DAILY effort to maintain a specified weight loss rate. On given days you may decide to take a walk or perform some other form of activity. On other days, you may decide to eat a light lunch. On some days you may decide to do both. But each day you must make a conscious effort to change. And the slope of your goal lines, the rate at which you want to lose weight, must be great enough to make daily changes NECESSARY. But don't over challenge yourself. You must take it SLOW and maintain your health.

What I am saying is that your upper goal line must be steep enough to challenge you but not so steep that there is difficulty in maintaining the weight loss rate. The lower goal line is a bit steeper and a bit more challenging. But the importance of the lower goal line is that it defines the maximum weight loss rate. For your health's sake, you do not want to go below the lower goal line. Your absolute goal is to stay inside the two goal lines.

If you are thinking, as you read this, about how fast you should lose the weight, think about this for a moment. Let's say you want to lose about 20 pounds. And let's say you are concerned about not wanting to make too many changes in your lifestyle. Say for example you're confined to a wheelchair and/or your ability to undertake activity is limited. Well, it's a simple trade off. If you want to make very few changes in your eating habits and maybe can't increase your physical activity, then it will take longer to lose the weight.

Let's say Ed is 64 years old and needs to shed 20 pounds. Let's say he weighs 210 and wants to get back down to 190. Because of Ed's age, his physical activities are limited and his job requires him to travel extensively. His choices in lifestyle modifications are limited. So he decides to just stop snacking in the evening. Because he's traveling, he can't weigh himself every day. But over the first month he lost almost two pounds. So, he figures if he continues this slight modification, he could possibly lose the twenty pounds over a year. That means by his retirement date he could be back to 190 pounds. Let's see … 20 pounds over 12 months, that's 20/12 = 1.67 or, 1 and 2/3 pounds per month. And to see how he's doing, he starts a graph and weighs himself as frequently as possible. And there's nothing wrong with this approach? Actually, it took Ed only about seven months to lose the excess weight. And he continued the practice and by his retirement date he had lost 25 pounds. So Ed was five pounds below his goal weight.

The reason I tell this story is to just emphasize that losing 20 pounds over a full year is just fine. There are those that will say. That's too long. I need to lose it quicker. Well, okay. That only means that to shorten the length of your journey (a quicker weight loss) you will have to make more lifestyle modifications. Which is the better approach? You have to make that decision. I will only say that the longer time period affords less dramatic changes and a better chance of continuing those lifestyle changes after the journey is over. And that means the person losing the weight over a longer period stands a better chance of keeping the weight off. That's why I keep harping on the "take it slow" approach. Look at this in a logical sense. If over a period of one year you stopped snacking in the evenings (and as a result you lost 20 pounds), don't you think it would be a simple process to continue that lifestyle in the months following that change in your diet, thus keeping the weight off (and possibly losing additional pounds in the subsequent months). Wouldn't it be wonderful if you had to <u>start</u> snacking on occasion to prevent getting too thin?

Now I mentioned just a few paragraphs ago that you must challenge yourself. I stated: "There is also the danger of not setting your goal high enough … If you decide to lose only a few pounds over an extended time period, you have not challenged yourself enough. You will, if you get on the scale each day and, over a period of ten days, see no weight loss; say to yourself, that's okay. I've got next week to lose a pound."

It may seem that I am now backtracking on that earlier statement. Actually I don't believe I have. The two approaches relate to two different situations. The first is that of the person who has a rather large amount of weight to shed, say 50 to 100 pounds. It can also be assumed that this person has a rather poor lifestyle that has gotten him or her into this situation. In this case there are probably some major changes needed in the lifestyle, both eating and activities. For this person, taking a slow approach lessens the chances of success. This person probably needs the challenge of multiple lifestyle changes.

The second situation is one of having to lose a smaller amount of weight. And because of the extenuating circumstances, a slow approach is okay. And since a single tactic (stop late evening snacking) is being employed, a longer period is perfectly all right.

You see, this is your journey. You set the rules. You do what is necessary to reach your objective. If you wanted to lose 120 pounds and decide to lose it at a rate of 2 pounds per month and you're happy with that and decide you're okay with taking five years to lose the weight, then that's great. Do whatever it takes for you to maintain the desired weight loss rate. There's always the danger that this slow approach doesn't present sufficient challenges. But if it works for you, go for it!

John Borntraeger

Chapter 8

FOOD CONTENT

Since we are talking about changing your eating habits, nutrition becomes extremely important. It is even more important if you are someone like me who doesn't eat (and doesn't like) the proper foods. Now this should not come as a surprise, but most people who need to lose weight do not eat a well balanced diet. Some people do eat properly. And if they find they need to lose some weight, they're probably not very active, or they are eating too much of the good things. But if you are like me, it is definitely a combination of eating and physical activity. I played sports when I was young. Baseball and tennis were the two sports I played and enjoyed. Yet, I remained overweight. And when I had spinal surgery, and could no longer play these sports, my size got completely out of hand.

There are a couple of general rules to help. Avoid, or reduce the amounts of, foods with high fat content. You might try drinking and cooking with 2% or 1% milk. Avoid large amounts of salt. Everything I am saying here, you hear daily on TV. You probably know what to avoid, and what you should be eating. But remember, this is not starting out as an exercise in denial. Modifications of your eating habits should be undertaken slowly. You and your doctor should be the ones who determine what changes you want to make, should make, and believe you are committed to, and able to make. But, at first, slow changes are the easiest to accomplish. More dramatic changes will come about later, but for surprisingly different reasons. We'll discuss that later.

I have only two recommendations. My first recommendation (and you should consult with your doctor on this) is to take a daily multivitamin if you're eating habits are as bad as mine. I did this at the insistence of my parents and doctor. And today, many years later, I still do. Any book on nutrition will tell what to eat and what to avoid. My second recommendation is to go to your bookstore or library and get a book on nutrition. Read it. Learn some things about your present diet and what changes would be helpful to an improved life.

You hear countless advertisements and see countless articles on fat content, calories, sugar, carbohydrates, saturated fats, unsaturated fats, trans-fats, and many other elements of our food and diet. What does all this mean? It means that we humans are beginning to be concerned about our diet. I'm not an expert on these topics and don't pretend to be. That is why I suggest you get some books on these topics, and talk to your doctor about these topics and how each affects you. Generally, you should, if you're overweight, limit your fat intake. This will also reduce your calorie intake. But remember, calories are energy. We need some calories to live. And, if you just reduce your fat and calorie intake and perform no physical activity, you could very well lose muscle.

You will find a great debate going on about the various types of "diets" out there. Some will tell you that the amount of fat you take in is of less concern than the amount of sugar. Some will say the carbohydrates and sugar are both of major concern because the carbohydrates turn to sugar once eaten. I will tell you this. There is a major increase in the number of diabetics in those countries where the diet has evolved to consuming large amounts of sugar and carbohydrates. You can go out and find a fat free food only to discover it is loaded with sugar. And that may be even more dangerous than the fat. I have read that it is estimated that we currently consume ten times more sugar than our grandparents consumed.

There is no doubt that these three elements of our diet are crucial to good health and critical in fighting the obesity that is prevalent in these countries. You will find in this great debate there are those that will tell you that the carbohydrate free diet is not healthy because we need some carbohydrates. And they're right. You do need some carbs (carbohydrates) in your diet. The problem is we are consuming way too many carbs. You will find those that say the amount of fat we take in is of little concern; the key is to take in protein and avoid sugar and carbs.

Guess what! I think they're all correct. We need to reduce the amount of fat we take in. We need to reduce the amount of sugar we take in. We need to reduce the amount of carbohydrates we take in. And now I will add my two cents worth. We also need to reduce the <u>quantity</u> of food we take in. We eat too much! We'll tackle that issue a bit later.

Now we've talked about all the bad stuff in our food; fat, sugar, carbs, etc. But shouldn't we talk about protein? The answer, of course, is yes. You need protein. Protein builds and maintains muscle. You don't need excessive carbohydrates. You don't need excessive fat. You don't need excessive sugar. You need to pay attention to the content of the foods you eat. How much of these items am I consuming? There are those that will tell you it is unhealthy to totally avoid carbohydrates, and sugar, and fat. And they're also right. Our problem in fighting obesity is that we don't moderate the amounts of these items. Limit your intake of those items that you know are unhealthy. Don't sit down and have a bowl of meatballs and spaghetti and consume eight pieces of bread with lots of margarine spread all over it. Have a little less spaghetti and only one piece of bread and limit the butter. Notice I said butter. Why? Avoid the trans-fats. In other words, when it comes to eating, we need to "get smart."

And read the labels on the food you eat: especially the snack foods. Get smart and start examining the content of the foods you eat. And as you modify the items you eat, based on the content (determined by reading the labels), examine your weight chart and you will find that the "smarter" you eat, the better your chances of staying inside your "weight envelope." There is an absolute link between the foods you eat and your weight. And that should not come as a surprise to anyone. But, it is this process that allows you to learn what to eat and what not to eat to achieve your weight-loss goal.

And I must once again emphasize this next point. Make absolutely certain that you are comfortable with the changes you are making. It is so very important that you remain comfortable with your lifestyle while working to change that lifestyle. This cannot and must not be a process where you deny yourself the foods you love. You can still eat the things you love.

You know, it comes down to this. How much do you love the "bad" things you eat versus how much do you love the new slimmer and healthy you. And again, you don't have to "give up" the bad, unhealthy things you love. You just have to learn moderation! You have to teach yourself to EAT SMART!

Chapter 9

WATER

I know this is a strange title for a chapter, and maybe to some even a strange topic. But water makes up for a rather large portion of our body weight. And, while I am on this topic, I will add one little footnote. And the topic of this footnote is salt. Though I have touched on this previously, a few additional comments are in order. Too much salt is not healthy. And it is known that salt makes the body retain water. And water is a heavy substance. And heavy substances in our body make us weigh more. Get the picture? By reducing the amount of salt we take in, we can have a remarkable effect on our body weight. And take notice that I used the word REDUCING. I didn't say to eliminate salt completely from your diet. I will continue to emphasize that this is not an exercise in denial. I couldn't live without salt. I love salt with my french fries. If I can't put salt on my eggs, I won't eat the eggs. And the same holds true for a good hamburger. Without salt, I don't want it. Okay, so much for the footnote on salt. Let's get back to the topic of water.

Many diets recommend that you drink a certain number of glasses of water each day. There are several reasons for this. Three reasons come to mind at this moment. One, it's healthy, and low in calories. Two, it helps to avoid hunger pains. A hunger pain is nothing more than the stomach contracting when there is nothing in it. Water will help to fill you up. Many diets recommend drinking a glass of water before a meal. You will tend to eat less. Boy! There's a novel idea. I wonder if I could lose weight by eating less. If this works for you, then that's great. The third reason is, to me, the most important. Drinking water helps to keep the body, and especially the kidneys, well flushed.

Stop and consider what takes place when we begin to lose weight. Body fat that was previously stored (and in my case most of it was stored near my navel) begins to melt away. Well, the word melt is a poor choice. What happens to this body fat when we lose weight? Well, first of all, body fat contains fluid. This fat is absorbed into the body and burned as calories. That's good. Since we are taking in fewer calories (hopefully), the body burns this fat. If we don't give the body some fat and calories through our mouth, then it goes and gets it from our waist. Isn't that great? The body really is a wonderful system. But it doesn't burn or consume all the elements of the fat. That portion that was fluid is passed on through our kidneys. But, this isn't the purest form of fluid. In fact, it is high in many substances that can be harmful. How harmful? Well, if you've ever had kidney stones, you know how harmful. Remember, in an earlier chapter, I related I had a bout with kidney stones in early March. In my experiences with diets, I have had an equal number of experiences with kidney stones. And that is (including spinal surgery) the most painful aliment I have ever suffered. I have been on several diets. And, usually associated with a New Year's resolution, I have always been on one of these diets, in the early months of the year. I have had four bouts with kidney stones. Each and every one has placed me in the hospital during the month of March. It wasn't until several years later that the link between my kidney stone problem was linked to my dieting.

The human body is made up of a large amount of water. It is this water that helps the body function in many ways. When we lose weight, the body goes through many changes. It is the additional water that assists the body in making these changes. Now I've already talked about the kidneys and the effects dieting can have on this organ and the need to stay hydrated during this journey. But now I'm going to talk about the gallbladder.

The gallbladder is a small pouch that stores bile. This bile is manufactured in the liver, and is released to assist the digestive process. When bile pigments, mineral salts, and other body products, form into hard stones in the gall bladder, the body is in for some horrible pain. In some cases, surgery for removal of these stones is necessary. And, in rare cases, gallstones can cause life-threatening complications. These stones are caused when the bile has high concentrations of cholesterol. Remember, this body fat that we are trying to lose just doesn't disappear. It must be absorbed by the body. And the body sometimes has difficulty absorbing it and getting rid of it. It is believed that dieting results in a shift in the balance of bile salts and cholesterol. The bile salts decrease and the cholesterol increases.

You can do three things to assist this process. <u>Number one</u>, and most important, you must lose the weight slowly. Losing weight rapidly, that is, utilizing a low calorie diet, results in a higher probability of developing gallstones. It is accepted that gallstones are a medically important complication of intentional weight loss. This is so, so very important. You have got to avoid rapid weight loss! You have got to go slowly.

<u>Number two</u>, drink plenty of water. Think of it as helping the body flush itself of this highly impure fat you have stored over the years. And <u>thirdly</u>, keep in touch with your physician before and during your lifestyle change program.

I mentioned earlier in this chapter that water helps the body function in many ways. Actually, help is not the proper word to describe the body's need for water. The proper word is depends. The body depends on water. The average adult is made up of 50 to 65% water. Water is necessary for the body's cells. Your organs need water. Your tissues need water. Water is necessary for temperature regulation. You joints need water for lubrication. We all know that thirst often results from higher temperatures. Increased activity also makes us thirsty. This thirst is simply the body's message to us that the level of fluids in our system is low. You can easily become dehydrated if you don't drink enough water. So, it's simple. Drink water when you're thirsty. And drink extra water when the temperature is high and when you are more active.

And here's one thing I experienced. In my case, dehydration resulted in a dull headache. And this brings up an extremely important point. Do not decide to decrease the amount of fluids you take in to increase your weight loss. This is a very dangerous idea. You will do damage to your body if you decrease your fluid intake.

So my recommendation to drink plenty of water comes with the utmost urgency. It helps keep the kidneys flushed, removing the impurities that result when the body begins to burn fat. It also helps to avoid hunger. And it quenches your thirst while adding zero calories to your daily intake. What more could you ask for? And it is <u>absolutely necessary</u> for bodily functions. Even if you are not on a diet or you're not trying to reduce your weight, doctors will tell you that you need to drink water. And most doctors will tell you that the vast majority of us do not drink enough water.

Chapter 10

THE ZONES

Now that you have made your graph, including your envelope (the red goal lines), it's time to think about how to stay inside those goal lines. What you will find, is that this task is the easiest in the beginning. Surprised? I didn't say it was easy in the beginning. I said it was the <u>easiest</u> in the beginning. You will get a better understanding of this statement in a few moments.

What you are going to experience in this journey can be broken up into three distinct areas, or time zones. The first will last a very short period of time; maybe five to ten days. This is the period where you will eat less or maybe just more intelligently, and increase your physical activity. Unfortunately, it is during this period that you may see fewer results. It is this starting period where only your commitment and the resulting good attitude can keep you on track. This first time zone is called the "start." Think of this as the period where you "start" the journey. The second period is the one I refer to as "the beginning." Think of this period as that in which you will "begin" to lose weight. It is a longer period. How long is impossible to say. It depends totally upon you. Each person is so different; there is no way to predict how long this period will last. Generally it will last longer for those people who need to lose more weight. And for some, this period lasts during the entire experience. They are the lucky ones. They never experience the third time zone. They are usually the people who have a well-balanced diet. Most of us, however, will experience this troublesome area or the third zone. I did. And I hope you do, for it is here that the learning experience takes place. We will discuss this third zone a little later. So, for now, let's get back to discussing "the start."

Physically, the first week to ten days can be difficult. This is where your commitment and attitude must keep you going. Why? Well, as I stated before, as you reduce your intake of high calorie food, the body has to burn fat (pounds) to make up for what it isn't getting through your mouth. This doesn't happen overnight. It will take time. How much time depends on you. And, again, it is important that you weigh yourself each and every morning to determine just how long it takes for you to start seeing the results. If you also undertake some additional activities, then the time necessary to see some results will be less, since you're burning calories at a higher rate. The reason for the importance of determining how long it takes to start seeing results is that it is an important clue. The longer it takes the more additional effort you must make to get started. Caution must be taken though! These additional efforts <u>must be gradual</u>. Don't stop eating completely, just to get started. It will have horrible consequences later. Understand that this process will take time. Don't push yourself too hard and too fast. Remember you are trying to form living habits that you are going to continue for the rest of your life. With this in mind, you can see how utterly stupid it would be to starve yourself just to get started. You can't continue that practice very long. And, this is so very important. Remember, you are forming a new way to live. Here, again is my graph for January, the first month.

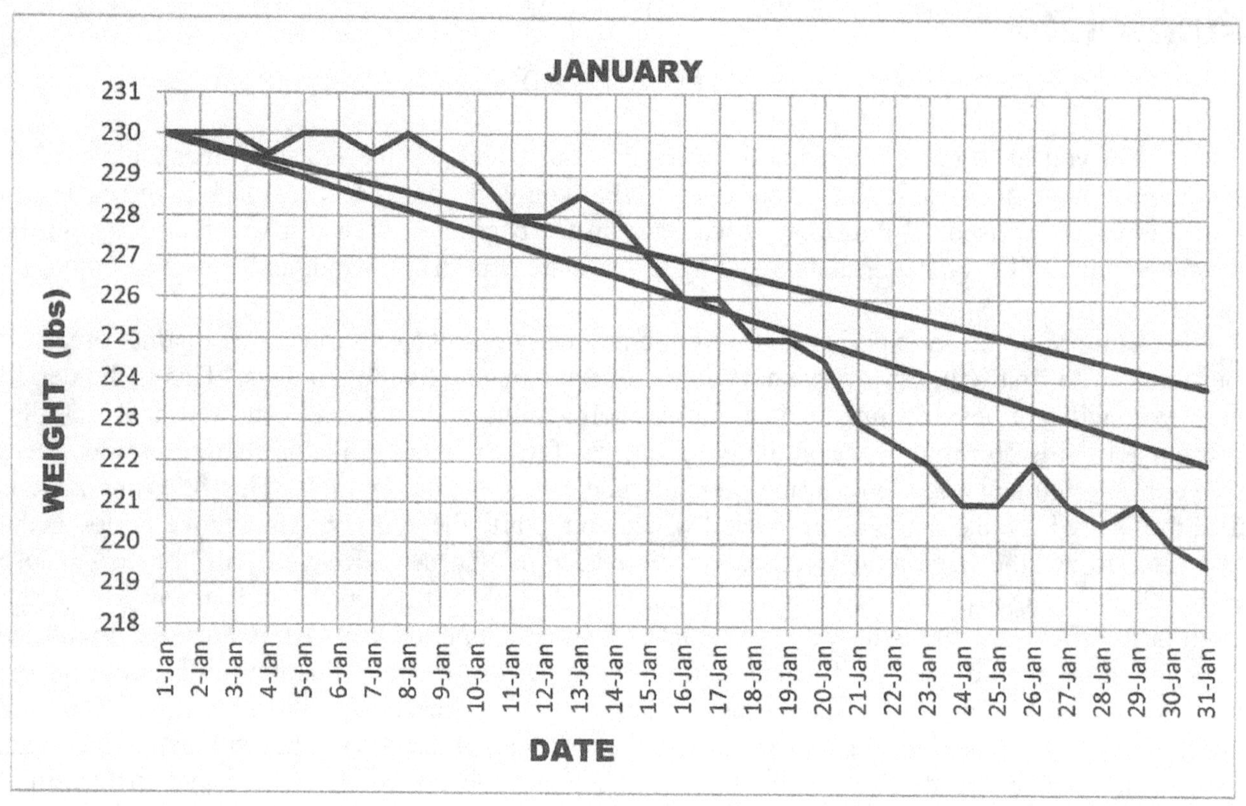

Notice that it took until January 10th to actually begin a downward slope. True, on January 4th one-half pound was lost, but the weight moved back and forth between 230 and 229 ½ for over a week. It was when the weight hit 229 that the "start" period was over and I was "beginning" to lose weight. I had moved into the second phase. So, my start phase lasted 9 days. Your start phase could be just a couple of days. It depends totally on you and what actions you take in eating smarter and doing some activity. I will offer one bit of advice. If you would like to minimize the length of the start zone, make a concerted effort to reduce your carbohydrates and sugar.

My start phase lasted a bit longer because I had been dependent on the pill to curb my appetite. On January 1st I stopped taking the appetite suppressants and without those pills, I was a bit hungrier and I was going back to my old ways of eating too much food. After all, I had been eating that way for years. It was only the pill that made me eat less. As I watched my graph and realized that I had stopped losing weight, as I had been when taking the pills, I became concerned, and I made a conscious effort to back off on the amount of food I was eating. And I specifically decided to try and lighten up on the amount of food I had for lunch. Within two days of this additional effort, I started dropping pounds once again.

Once this process starts, you will begin to see the pounds disappear. This marks the end of the "start" zone. You have now entered the zone I call the "beginning." This is the easiest time zone. Why? Well, now you will begin to see results. You will begin losing pounds, and as you see results, your enthusiasm keeps you going. Your attitude gets better, and it is much, much easier to continue with the minor modifications you have made to your eating habits and physical activity habits.

Look again at my January graph and you will see that by January 15th I was back inside my envelope and on January 18th I actually dropped below the envelope and continued to lose pounds at a rate faster than I had hoped for. By the end of January, I had lost an additional ten and one-half pounds. And believe me I was happier about losing those ten plus pounds than I was about the many pounds I had lost in the previous three months. Why? Because this graph was the first concrete evidence that I was able to do this. And I was doing it without the help of the appetite suppressant pills. For the first time in my life I knew I was in control. I was making this happen. I was finally able to lose weight; something I had wanted to do for years. And I did it in one month. I was losing weight at a rate faster than I had hoped and faster than in the previous three months. And I was enjoying it and I was not miserable because I never stopped eating the things I loved. I realized I was eating smarter. I was still eating the items I love, just eating less of those items.

At this point I was thinking how easy this was and how I was going to hit my goal weight much faster than I had hoped. But, I was in for a surprise. I was about to hit the third zone. And I'm sure you will discover this third zone as well. It is here that you begin to learn a great deal more about yourself. It is where the education begins. It is where you really begin to take control of your weight.

Note that on January 31st I hit 219 ½ pounds. Then on February 1st I weighed 220 pounds. And it was there that I stopped losing weight.

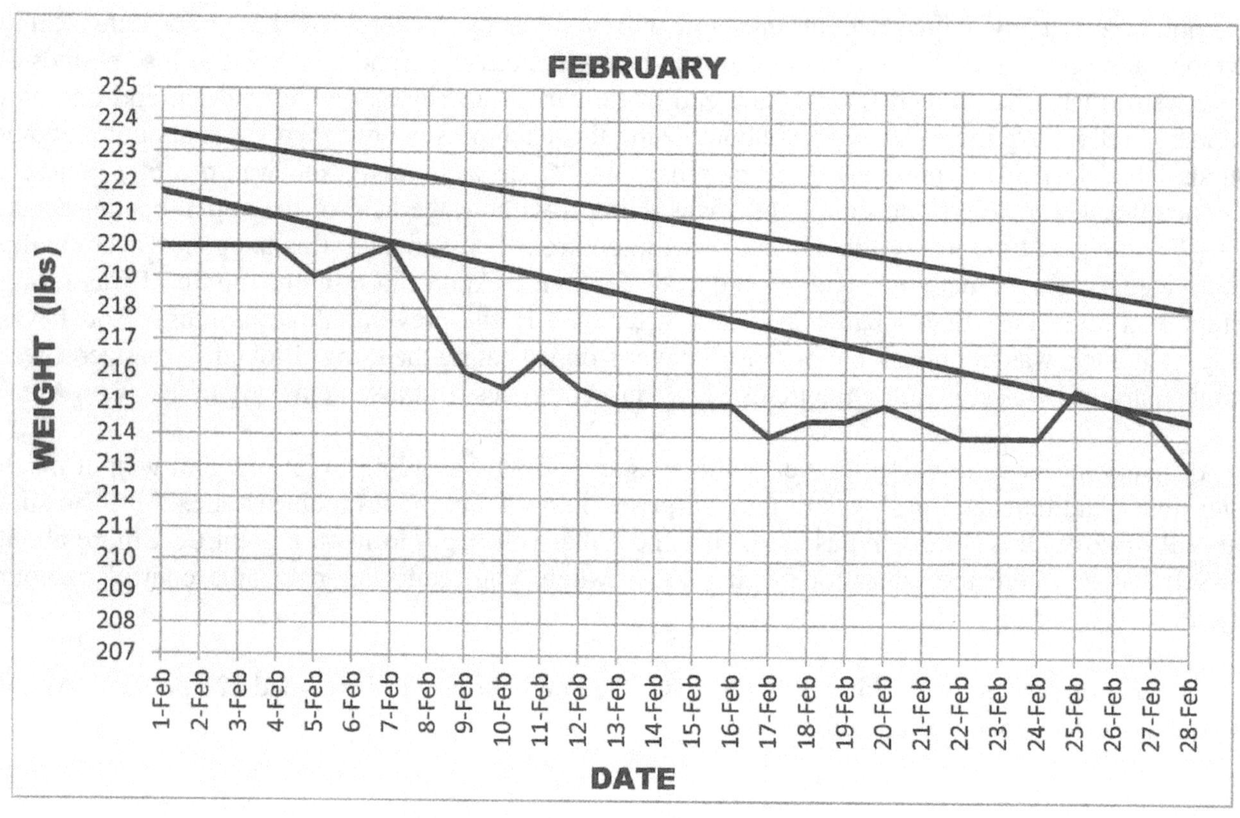

And for four days my weight stayed at 220. I couldn't figure out what had happened. Then on the 5th of February I dipped down to 219. Then on the next day back up again. I was amazed that all of a sudden I stopped losing weight and could not figure out why. So, on the 6th and 7th of February, I ate a bit less and made sure I walked. I couldn't play golf because it was just too cold, but I did take a walk at lunch for those two days. And then on the morning of Feb 8th, I started the downward trend again.

After a certain amount of time (and how long differs for each person), you will see the rate at which pounds disappear begin to drop off. In other words, the number of pounds lost per week will decrease. In fact, as happened to me in early February, you may find that you are no longer losing weight. When this happens, welcome to the world of the plateau. "Plateau" is a word of french origin meaning a flat area. This term is used in geography to describe a flat area found in mountainous country. This is the third zone. And you will probably hit many plateaus.

Though I will discuss these areas in a later chapter, a few comments are in order. It is these troublesome areas where you begin to learn something about your living habits. It is also because of these flat spots that you really begin to change your living habits. The education begins here. Believe it or not, these flat spots are the best thing about this technique. They are sort of a blessing in disguise. It is because of these times when you stop losing the pounds that you have to determine why it has happened, and how to get off of this flat spot, and get started on a downward slope again.

An even greater lesson will be learned if at some point, and I guarantee this will happen to you, you find that on some morning you get on the scale, and BINGO, you've gained two pounds, or you gained one pound on each of two or three consecutive days.

And here is another good reason for weighing yourself every morning. Let's imagine you are on some other kind of "diet," and you weigh yourself only once each week. Say you weigh yourself every Friday afternoon. And all during the week you really work hard on this imaginary diet. But on weekends your willpower fails, and you go out each Friday and or Saturday night and really "put on the bag." Each Friday afternoon (before you go out for the weekend), you weigh yourself and find that you have lost one pound. That's great. But what you are NOT doing is changing your living habits. You're dieting! And you're dieting only five days a week! This doesn't bother you, because you're losing weight. If you were weighing yourself daily, you would see the negative aspects of these Friday and Saturday night "binges." It is only through discovering these moments of weakness that you have the opportunity to do something about them. If you had known the negative effects of these "weakends," you may have been able to lose two pounds each week instead of just one pound. Notice that I spelled weekend as "weakend." I use the "ea" rather then the "ee" because it seems to be the period where it is the most difficult to maintain lifestyle changes. We tend to fall back into old habits on "weakends."

Hopefully this will explain why it is so important to weigh yourself each and every morning, as soon as you awake. It gives you the opportunity to discover the consequences of those periods where we fall back into old habits and to analyze what we did to ourselves. Then, and only then, will we possibly avoid doing it again next "weakend."

And while I am "harping" on this topic, the person in the above scenario is only kidding himself or herself. And they are not treating their body as well as they should. What you will find out, is that these "binges" take an enormous toll on your effort to slim down. Now don't start worrying that you won't be able to wander on occasion, and enjoy yourself at a party or some other social gathering. You will! But you will learn to moderate your food intake at these events. Why? Well, you will learn the consequences of overdoing it. In fact, it is almost mandatory that you DO go on a binge at some point during this experience, and I probably won't have to order you to do it. Most all of us do this on occasion and it's quite natural. But you are going to learn from the experience. You will learn the cost of such behavior, and will have to decide for yourself whether or not it's worth it.

And here's one additional point. In chapter nine I talked about water and the importance of drinking sufficient amounts of water. Water and a high intake of sodium (salt), which promotes water retention, can have a major influence on your weight on any given day. But do not stop drinking water to ensure you lose weight tomorrow or as an attempt to get off a plateau. Insufficient water can have a catastrophic result. But do try to minimize or reduce the amount of salt you consume.

Chapter 11

DAILY WEIGHING

I have talked several times about the necessity of weighing yourself every day. Now I realize that not everyone has a scale. But this daily weighing is so very important. If you don't have a scale, you must purchase or borrow one. It is critical to the success of the journey.

Now I know that all of the "diet" experts are going to take off on this statement. But daily weighing IS important. What others will tell you is that what you weigh this morning is collectively affected by the food intake and amount of physical activity of many previous days. And that yesterday's intake and activity is the least important. In other words, if you weigh yourself on Friday, they will tell you that the days closest to Friday have the least influence on your weight.   They will insist that you should look collectively at the 7 days prior to weighing.

I disagree with this. In fact, you will find the amount of food you ate yesterday will have a profound effect on today's weight. I think it is important to detect any trends as soon as possible. The reason for this urgency is due to the importance of trying to relate the trend to the cause.   It's a bit difficult to follow what I'm about to say without a visual aid.   So I'll provide this calendar to help.

SUN	MON	TUES	WED	THURS	FRI	SAT
No Activity		Extra Lasagna		No Activity	Weigh-in	

If, for example, you had no physical activity on Sunday and Thursday, and had an extra helping of Lasagna on Tuesday, what affect did each have on your weight taken on Friday? It's impossible to say. If you had been weighing yourself daily, you may have seen your weight loss rate fluctuate on each day, and have had the chance to relate that fluctuation to what and how much you ate on those days and the activity or lack of activity of the one or two days prior. Let's assume you have been walking each day for about 15 minutes, and have been reducing the amount of high calorie foods you eat. Let's also assume you weigh 144 pounds, and have been losing about ten pounds per month. Now that's an excessive and dangerous amount of weight to lose in one month. I'm using 10 pounds only as a round number to explain this concept. That means you are losing about one pound every three days. By noting that on Monday and Tuesday morning your weight remained constant, you have seen the results of the lack of physical activity on Sunday. And just maybe, knowing this, you wouldn't eat that second helping on Lasagna at dinner on Tuesday. And if you did eat the Lasagna on Tuesday, you will probably be shocked to see that you have gained a pound if you weigh yourself on Wednesday morning. And, due to your lack of activity on Thursday, that pound gained will probably still be around on Friday and Saturday.   You have just seen the price paid for the extra helping of lasagna and the lack of activity on Sunday and Thursday. Now, when you weighed yourself on Thursday morning and saw that your weight loss had stopped or maybe even gained a pound because of Sunday's lack of activity and Tuesday's extra helping of Lasagna, I would hope that your commitment to yourself and your improving health would influence you to decide to take that walk on Thursday.   And just maybe, you would walk a little further. Are you beginning to see how you can slowly change your lifestyle to live a healthier life? It's all a question of being in control.

At some other time during this experience you will note days when you weren't able to maintain your physical activity, but due to your conscious efforts in watching what you eat, did in fact maintain a gradual weight loss. This is the educational aspect of this whole technique. This is so important, and I can't emphasize this enough. It is absolutely necessary for you to relate what you are doing and eating to how it affects your weight EVERY SINGLE DAY. If you have been losing at a relatively constant rate, then all of a sudden, you stop losing, try and relate this back to your activity (eating and physical activity) over the past few days. Teach yourself what you need to do to maintain that gradual weight loss rate. If, on a given day, the weather is beautiful and you take a second 15 minute walk in the evening, watch your weight and see if it has a positive influence. If you go to a party and have more to eat than you feel was normal, watch your weight, and see how long it will take to get back to the rate of weight loss you had before going to the party. What you may find, is that it will take you maybe as much as ten days to get back to the same weight loss rate. If this happens, and the next time you go to a party, or are offered a second helping of lasagna, you'll remember this experience and refuse to over-indulge. You have taught yourself a lesson. You have begun to modify your life-style. If you find yourself thinking, "Let's see ... if I take a second helping of lasagna, then I will have to walk TWICE a day for three days to maintain my current weight loss rate." You are learning to be in control of your life. And that is what this technique is all about. You CAN teach yourself to be in control of your life.

But the only way to do this is to weigh yourself every single day, and relate this weight and weight loss rate to your recent activity. At this point I am going to relate a few of my experiences. First of all, I love breakfast. It is the one meal I wouldn't miss for the world. And, while I'm talking about meals, here's an important statement. I never skip a meal! Don't try this. Eat three meals a day. You may, as I did on occasion, establish one of these meals as a light meal. But I always eat three meals. Getting back to my breakfast, I did modify the foods I eat at breakfast. I have two eggs, fried in real butter rather than margarine, and at first I had one piece of whole wheat toast rather than my usual two pieces of white bread/toast. Now, I don't eat the toast at all. I eat just the eggs. And sometimes I'll have one strip of bacon. Not six pieces of bacon; just one. Very seldom do I eat anything else with my eggs. Sometimes I have cereal with 1% milk instead of eggs. I love eggs, but my intelligent eating habits are aware of the need to monitor my cholesterol intake. But now that's changed. Now they are saying the egg is the perfect food. And for lunch I try to eat very light. I decided that lunch was the one meal where I could make the biggest changes. For lunch I would have a soda (soft-drink in some areas of the country) and a package of peanut-butter crackers. Oh, do I have a weakness for peanut-butter. Or maybe I'll have a hard boiled egg. And I try to take a twenty to thirty minute walk every day just before or after lunch. And what do I do about my dinner? Well, I usually eat a normal dinner. If I had more than usual for lunch, I may eat a light dinner. But I am always aware of the quality and quantity of what I am eating and how it will affect my weight tomorrow morning and the mornings to follow.

I'm going to go back and talk a bit about the gallbladder. Here's another reason to avoid skipping meals. When you skip meals, you decrease the gallbladder contractions. And if the gallbladder doesn't contract and empty out the bile, stones can begin to form due to the concentrations of cholesterol in the bile that may result from your dietary changes. So, DO NOT SKIP MEALS! The results can be dangerous to your health.

Now, let's get back to our subject. It's strange what we can do if we set our minds to it. I mentioned that I had a soda or soft-drink with lunch. There was a time when I could not stand the taste, or after taste, of diet drinks. But when I set my mind to it, it took only two weeks to cultivate a taste for the diet drinks. Now, if a waitress mistakenly beings a non-diet drink, I couldn't drink it if I wanted too. It's just too sweet. Again, intelligence has dictated a healthier eating habit. It is just one additional change I decided to make for me to continue losing weight. Again it is an issue of being in control of your life and your choices. And weighing yourself every day and seeing the positive and negative affects of these choices helps you to make better choices.

And here's an additional thought about the lunch. Yes. Peanut butter is high in sugar, and it is fattening. But it is also very high in protein. And yes the crackers are very high in carbs. Would a lunch of some meatballs with swiss cheese be better? There are very few carbs in the meatballs and cheese. The answer is probably yes. That's a low carb high protein meal. And sometimes that is precisely what I have for lunch. But it is also high in fat and too much cheese can elevate your cholesterol. So I don't eat that for lunch every day. And when I have either the meatballs or the peanut butter, or a hard boiled egg, the amount I eat is a moderate amount. You see, you must determine what works best for you. You must weigh all these factors and determine what works for you. As I mentioned before, I love peanut butter. And though the package of crackers and peanut butter is not the most wholesome lunch ever, I love it, and the total number of calories consumed was far less than what I had previously been eating for lunch; namely two hamburgers, a big order of fries, and a large cola, loaded with sugar. Get the point?

And here is another topic that is worth mentioning. It is the topic of quality versus quantity. And again, the "experts" will probably take issue with me on this. First, we all agree (even the experts) that quality is very important. What you eat does have a major impact on your weight. But, and here is where some will argue, quantity IS important. But it's not important for everyone. Those people who are able to maintain a very healthy, and well balanced diet, and who maintain a healthy activity schedule, don't have to worry about quantity. I doubt very seriously if they will even read this. Why should they? They don't have to worry about their life-style. But those of us, who do have to worry, and work at keeping a healthy weight, should be concerned with the quantity of food we take in. This of course is not our only concern. We must be concerned with the quality of our food, as well. But, it is my contention, that we should try and reduce the quantity of food we eat. This is precisely the point of the peanut butter crackers for lunch instead of the burgers and fries. What food should we be concerned with in terms of quantities? Well, I doubt if I really have to list those foods where we need to reduce the amount or quantity we consume.

If you were to sit down for dinner at Aunt Gertrude's house and had the following choices, what, and how much of each would you eat? Good ole' "Aunt Gerty" has placed before us mashed potatoes, broccoli, corn on the cob, her famous potato rolls, and corn muffins, baked chicken, and her equally famous lasagna, and a bowl of spaghetti. You see her husband, Uncle Leonard, is Italian, and he must have Italian food at every meal. Oh, and she's also prepared two fresh water trout (broiled) that nephew Steve caught in the lake this morning.

The question is what would you choose and how much would you eat? I know at one time, I would have lasagna (at least two helpings), several rolls smothered in lots of margarine. And I'd probably have a corn muffing or two, also smothered in margarine. And I guarantee I will eat whatever she has for desert and maybe even two helpings. Now, since I have passed up the corn, broccoli, baked chicken, and broiled fish, you will never convince me that the amount of food I consumed has no bearing on my weight. My contention is that those of us who are overweight got this way by eating too much of the wrong things. And one thing we must do is to reduce the amount of these types of foods. Especially since I am not advising you to avoid these foods, you must AT LEAST reduce the quantity. Remember, this is not an exercise in denial. Denial of those things we love will make this a horrible experience, and in all probability, therefore, a failure.

I can recall one incident in the early days of my attempt to lose weight through the use of this graph. It happened in early April. I've included my April graph to demonstrate the results of overindulging.

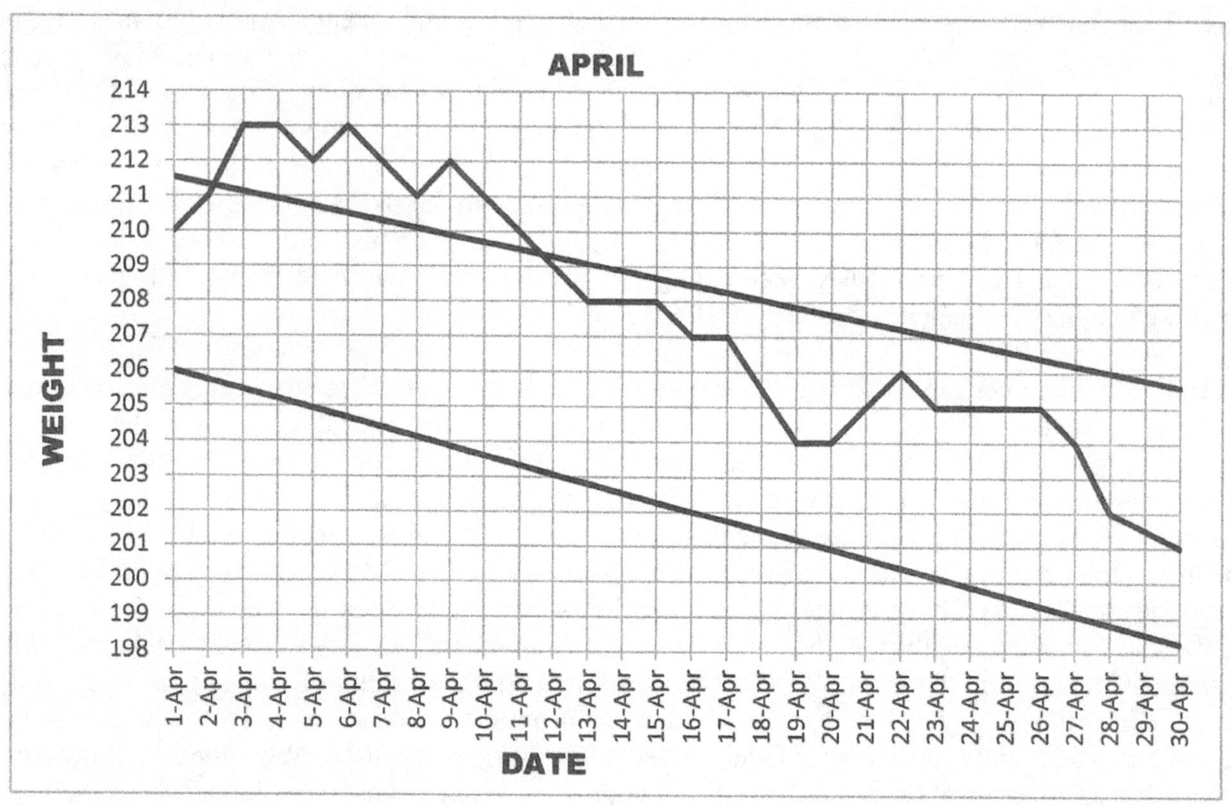

I had gone through the month of March and had only lost about three pounds but was finally starting a down trend. I had lost about 20 pounds using the graph and was feeling really good about myself and my efforts. About 2 days after I started on a downward slope again, I had a lasagna dinner that could have fed three people. The next morning, April 3rd, I got on my scale and found I had put on two pounds. I thought, "That's ok, it is just a temporary set-back." "My weight will be back where it was tomorrow." Brother! I was in for one major surprise.

Chapter 12

BINGES

We have all heard the saying, "all work and no play makes Jack a dull boy." Well, the same holds true for an effort to change our body weight through changing our lifestyle. "All work and denial makes Jack miserable." You are going to go through periods where your willpower and commitment fail you. But please don't let this discourage you. Learn from it. View it as part of your education. It is an experience you must go through. It is an important experience for two reasons. First, you must experience what it will take to recover from this binge. You must experience the efforts necessary to get your weight and rate of weight loss back to where it was prior to the binge. And second, since this lesson will stay with you, you can avoid this happening again. The concept of this NOT being a process of denial holds true for all aspects of our life. We will still have to go to parties, and will definitely have to go to many more dinners at Aunt Gertrude's. But we can even learn to control our binges. Experience is still the best teacher around.

The episode I related in the previous chapter was my first experience of going outside my envelope. I had been losing weight at a good rate. I was absolutely tickled with myself. Then I hit the flat spot or plateau in mid March. I was getting dangerously close to the upper goal line. I made a few changes in diet and level of activity and the downward slope began once again in late March. Then I celebrated with that April 2nd lasagna dinner. What a disaster! Not only did I gain two pounds, but I also crossed the upper goal line. For the first time I was outside my envelope. I was in danger of not making my goal weight. I continued my increased level of activity, and tried to cautiously watch what I was eating. It took six days to lose those two pounds, and another three days to get a downward slope started again. And, it was another day to get back inside my envelope. That huge lasagna dinner was a costly experience. It took ten days to recover from this moment of excessive eating. But I did learn my lesson. In fact, the exact same day I got back inside the envelope, we had lasagna for dinner that night.

And what did the experience teach me. Well, I had one half of what I usually eat, and about one fourth of what I had that famous night. And I was absolutely amazed that I wasn't hungry later that night. The portion I had eaten was more than sufficient. In essence, I discovered that the helping I had been eating for all these years was too much. I had no way of knowing that. I love lasagna. I had been eating that amount for years because I love it, and not because I needed it. The lesson I learned was that I loved what was happening to my appearance more than I loved the lasagna. And what happened the next morning? Well, my downward slope continued.

And here's another good example of the positive aspect of daily weighing. Let's say that on Monday you have a double serving of meatballs and spaghetti and three or four slices of Italian bread, with margarine, of course. Next morning (Tuesday) you weigh and have gained 1 pound. You had been losing a ½ pound every two or three days and now that has stopped. Eventually (maybe three or four days later), you get back to losing an average of ½ pound every two or three days. Then your wife serves-up meatballs and spaghetti again or your husband takes you to Benito's Italian Restaurant. This time you eat ½ as much as the previous time and the next morning you find that you didn't gain the 1 pound as earlier experienced. And you find that you didn't experience starvation before the next morning's breakfast. The point is, if you watch your daily weight and rate of weight loss and relate it to your daily eating and activities, you will begin to realize you're eating more than you need.

This is just one example of how relating your weight each day to the previous day's activities can be such a learning experience. If you were weighing yourself only once per week, there would be no way of knowing the negative aspects of this over-indulgence or relating the effects of these two separate meals on your weight

So don't think this method of weight reduction through changing your lifestyle has any rules about binges. It doesn't. Parties and special dinners at Aunt Gertrude's are all part of our lives. We must continue to go to these events. But we must learn to control our lifestyle (eating) at all times, even at these special events. When we can do this, it just becomes part of our daily life and not a binge.

Chapter 13

PLATEAUS

It may seem repetitive to have a chapter on plateaus since we have already covered many of the aspects of this troublesome time where the weight loss stops for whatever reason. But it is extremely important to concentrate on this topic and discuss it in greater depth for two reasons.

MULTIPLE PLATEAUS

First, you will probably experience more than one plateau. In fact, you'll probably experience multiple plateaus. And each time not only could the cause of the plateau be different, but a different technique may and should be required to get off the plateau. In other words, what worked the first time may not be effective the second time. And that shouldn't come as a surprise if you stop and think about. You should be continuing the activities that got you off a previous plateau. In other words, when you hit a plateau and you change either your eating habits or your activities to get off that plateau, you must continue with the newly modified lifestyle. If you don't continue those lifestyle changes, I guarantee your weight loss will stop again.

Let's look at this in greater detail. Your weight loss rate goes to zero. And let's say you decide that instead of having late night snacks every night, you have them every other night. And in a couple of days, you start losing weight again. If you went back to having snacks every night just after the weight loss resumed, you haven't accomplished a positive change in your lifestyle and I can guarantee you will quickly experience another plateau. So the lifestyle changes must be continued. And, I'll repeat this again. This is the reason your lifestyle changes must be small ones that you can easily accept and endure. And, I'll also repeat the words, "This must be a pleasant experience." It must not be one of denying yourself a lifestyle that's necessary for your happiness.

So, if you do in fact continue having fewer late night snacks and in a couple of weeks you experience another plateau, it's time to do some more lifestyle changes. Maybe you can go to snacking every third night. Try different things and determine what works for you.

DANGEROUS CONSEQUENCES

And the second reason for an expanded discussion on the topic of plateaus is the most important. When multiple plateaus are experienced (and some find that each subsequent plateau is a bit more difficult to exit than the previous) we can lose enthusiasm, and our attitude and commitment weaken. For these two reasons I am going to discuss all the aspects of this sometime troublesome period and concentrate on effectively exiting a plateau as quickly as possible before we "lose heart."

There are actually three aspects of the plateau that we must consider. First, the cause, and second, the remedy, or the way to get a downward slope started again. And the third aspect is, as stated above, that for some people it can be the reason there journey halts and the weight loss stops. Plateaus can cause some to give up on the process and fail to successfully change their lifestyle.

THE CAUSE

The cause or reason our rate of weight loss has stopped is important in that it teaches a lesson. It makes us aware of various activities or lack of activities that may have caused the plateau. Children often wonder why they study history. Simply put, one reason is it teaches what not to do in the future. The causes of a flat spot, or sudden halt in our downward slope, are many. The first usually signals the end of that zone I called the beginning. You will recall that I mentioned it is important to weigh yourself every day. It is only through daily weighing that you can determine that you are on a plateau. I mentioned previously that during the "beginning" period, your body is burning up the fat stored in your body. And during this period, your weight loss can be rather drastic and rapid. But, like all good things, this will come to an end. When it does, you will have hit your first plateau.

Now since few of us will have a scale that can indicate fractions of a pound, we will have to discuss what actually constitutes a plateau. If you have been losing weight at a rate of 5 pounds per month, then you're losing about 1/2 pound every three days. Under these conditions, a plateau could be defined as a period of six days without any weight loss. Your weight could actually fluctuate up or down 1 or 2 two pounds. But generally you will experience a period where your net loss will be zero pounds over a period of 6 to 10 days.

Okay. So now we know what a plateau is and how to recognize it. But what causes it. Well, there are probably unlimited reasons or explanations as to why it occurs. It could be a physical thing. For some reason every person I know who has lost weight on diets and every single person who has lost weight through this technique have all said that once they started losing weight they lost a large amount of weight for the first month or so and then their rate of weight loss slowed down. To prove the point, take a look at the graph of my weight from January 1st through March 31st.

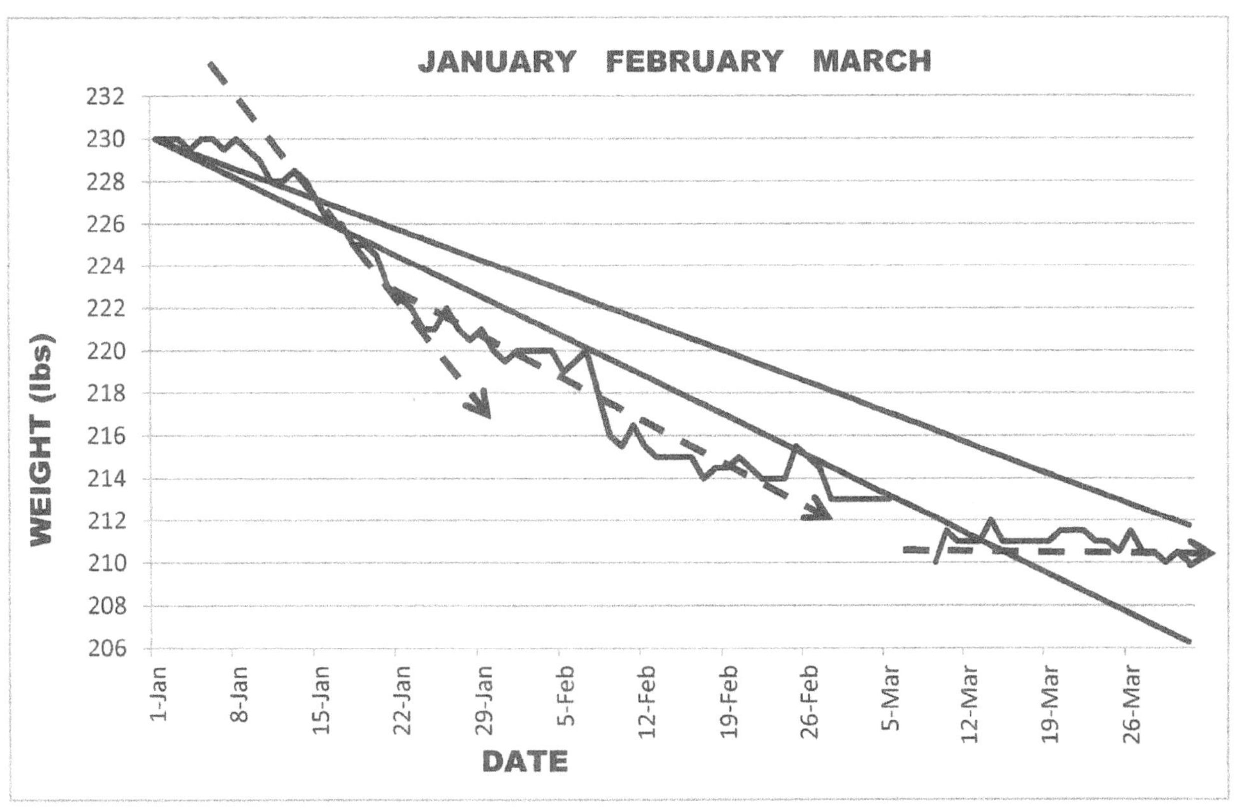

Once I began losing weight (January 10th), the weight loss rate was about four pounds a week until about January 25th. Then, the rate slowed down to about 2 pounds a week. Then about March 10th, it came to a halt and didn't start again until about March 25th. I've drawn three dashed lines on the graph to show the rate of weight loss during these three periods. Also note that the rate from late January to early March was just about equal to the lower goal line. The two lines are parallel, meaning the lower goal weight loss rate and the weight loss rates for February are just about equal, 1.9 pounds per week, or half of what it was in January. Why the change? Nobody knows for sure. It could be that I was feeling comfortable about the weight loss and was getting slack in my attention to what I was eating and how much. Maybe due to the weather, I wasn't walking as often.

Plateaus are the same way. My weight loss rate changed between January and February. Who knows why? And though we care why this has happened, it is more important to detect the change. We care that we have noticed the decrease in the rate at which weight is lost. We care because once detected, we can change our lifestyle to compensate. My weight loss rate also changed between February and March. Except in the case of a plateau, the weight loss rate goes from some acceptable rate to zero pounds lost. Plateaus can be, and usually are, caused by changes in eating habits (both amounts and quality); activity changes, and believe it or not, changes in your sleeping habits. I'm not sure why they happen. And what's more, who cares. The fact is it will happen to you. If you suspect that you have hit a plateau or the rate of weight loss begins to decrease, for one of the above reasons, then avoid that pitfall. It reminds me of the old joke where a guy goes to his doctor, moves his arm a certain way and says to the doctor, "Doctor, it hurts when I do this." And the doctor replies, "Then don't do that." Same thing applies here. If you suspect you know what caused the plateau, learn from the experience and avoid doing that in the future. It is part of the learning experience. It is how you take control of your lifestyle.

Now I know it sounds a bit contradictive to say "who cares" when I talked above about why weight loss stops. But consider these two scenarios. And both will occur while you are on this journey. First case: You are losing weight at about 1.5 pounds per week. And you take a trip or it rains for five consecutive days. You weight loss stops and you go two weeks and gain almost two pounds. What caused the weight loss rate to stop and caused you to gain almost two pounds. That one is, as they say, a "no brainer."

But what if you didn't change a thing in your activity and also didn't change any of your eating habits. There is the possibility that you will have changed nothing in your activity and eating habits, yet your rate of pounds lost per week begins to decrease, or in the case of a plateau, your pounds lost rate goes to zero. What happened here? Well, we don't know. And here is where the phrase "who cares" applies. No one knows why this happens. It just happens. And when you realize it is happening to you, it's time to make some more (small) changes. And I emphasize "small" again to ensure you, first, make this experience a pleasant one (don't quit eating for two days), and second, it is important that if and when you get off this plateau you know what helped. So, you might even consider only trying one additional change in lifestyle. For example, change from having bread at every meal to only two or three nights a week. It is very hard to relate a weight loss rate change to multiple changes in lifestyle.

I am certain from my experience and that of many others who have utilized this technique of changing their lifestyle or losing weight on any diet, there comes a point where you have to do a bit more than you did at the outset. I believe that one of the reasons that the early weight loss rate is a bit higher is that during the first several weeks of this process, you tend to rid your body of excess fluid. There really isn't anything bad about this process. It is a good thing. But it does emphasize the importance of drinking plenty of water. Keep your kidneys flushed!

But again, it doesn't really matter why this is happening. What does matter is that you are weighing yourself every day and recognize it is happening and do something about it so you don't get near and go over your upper goal line.

Whatever the cause, you will find that your weight loss will probably be most dramatic in the beginning phase. Your rate of pounds lost per week will lessen and you will hit plateaus. What can you do to increase your rate of weight loss when you hit this next zone? Well, I think the answer is rather obvious. You are going to have to make some additional changes in your living habits, both eating and physical activity.

This whole process is like a staircase. Each time you get off of a plateau, by increasing your physical activity and watching what you eat, along comes another plateau. In other words, the longer you work at this, the more changes you must make. Actually it isn't more difficult. It just takes additional amounts of effort on your part to maintain a weight loss rate so that you can achieve your goal. You could view this as attacking layers of fat stored in our body. Once we burn off one layer, we have to attack the next layer with a little more zest.

Now, please don't get alarmed at the prospect of this whole process getting tougher as you go along. It really isn't that difficult. What you will find is that this becomes more of a challenge than anything. You are seeing good results, your happy with your success, and BINGO, you hit a plateau. Getting off that plateau is more of a challenge than a chore. And believe me, what you will learn about yourself and what you can do is worth a million dollars. And here lies the beauty of this whole process. At each plateau, you make a tiny additional effort. And hopefully you will continue to make these tiny efforts. And in the end, these tiny efforts will add up to a major change in your lifestyle. You will have learned very slowly to do what it takes to change your body through changing your lifestyle. You will learn not only what it takes to lose weight, but you will have gradually changed your living habits and that will enable you to keep the weight off.

There can be other reasons for plateaus. You may find that you go on a business trip and have a difficult time monitoring what you eat. I know when I went on one of these business trips, it was sometimes disastrous. So, you're gone for three or four days. You come back and find that you didn't lose a single pound while gone, and may in fact have gained a little. Another reason may be that while you were away, you couldn't maintain the level of physical activity you were performing. Or, you may be at home and it rains for three days straight. And because of this, you couldn't take your usual walk or play golf. Or maybe you were forced by Aunt Gertrude to have a second piece of her lasagna, and two pieces of her famous pecan pie. After all, you can't insult Aunt Gertrude. All of these things could halt the rate at which you have been losing weight. The important thing here is to recognize, if you can, what caused the plateau. You may even want to record on your graph the number of minutes of activity each day, or indicate what physical activity you performed each day. You may also want to place on your graph, some indication of the amount of food you ate each day. For example, you could put a red dot at the bottom of your graph on those days when you ate more than usual, a yellow dot on those days when you ate an average amount of food, and a green dot on those days when you ate less than your normal amounts. I can guarantee you will begin to see a relationship between the rate of weight loss (and plateaus) and the amount of food you eat and your activity levels. And this relationship should not come as a surprise. In a later chapter we will talk about calories. If you take in more calories than you expend (activity) you will gain weight. And if you expend more calories than you take in you will lose weight. It's the same as in finance. If you spend more money than you make, you're in trouble.

But, as I said before, you will hit plateaus and have no clue as to why your weight loss rate stopped. Okay. In this case, just accept that sometimes we don't know what causes the plateau. Accept it as a fact of life and do what is necessary to get off the plateau and start your weight loss trend.

So, if you know what caused the plateau, that's great. Learn from it. If you don't know what caused the plateau, don't lose any sleep over it. In both cases, just do what is necessary to get started on your downward trend.

What you will learn about yourself will astonish you. I know of a minister who became so good at this that it became a game with him. Over a period of two months, he proved that he could actually predict when a plateau was going to occur and could do something to prevent it. What he noticed was that he hit a plateau just about every Tuesday. Could it be that famous culprit, "weakend?" Regardless of why it was happening, he found that by playing 9 holes of golf on Sunday evening, he would not experience a plateau on Tuesday. To prove his point, he played 9 holes of golf every other Sunday. And for two months he found that he would hit a plateau only on those Tuesdays following a Sunday on which he did not play golf. If he played some weekend golf, his weight loss rate would continue right on through the week.

Okay. So a plateau could be caused by many things. It may be overeating, or decreased physical activity, or it may be something you can't figure out. Usually, you will be able to determine a cause. But occasionally, you won't have a clue. In this case, it is probably something going on in your body. It could be a change in your metabolic make-up. I honestly think that as your body changes, and believe me it does go through some changes when you lose weight, the rate at which the body burns fat actually changes at times. Whatever the cause, it is important to recognize a plateau and understand that it doesn't have to signal the end of your efforts. It is also important to recognize it quickly. If it goes on for several days, you could be in danger of going outside (above) your envelope.

And, as we age, we lose some of the calorie-burning muscle. And between the ages of 30 and 50, due to metabolic changes we will burn 200 less calories performing the same activity.

THE REMEDY

Okay. So now we know how to recognize a plateau. And, in most cases, we know what causes it, and will therefore try to avoid it. But it is going to happen to you. So, what do we do once we realize we have stopped losing weight at the rate we want? Well, there are two obvious answers and a couple of not so obvious answers. First, the obvious ones are increase your activity level, and/or more closely monitor the quantity and quality of the food you eat. Maybe even cut back on your snacking. Or instead of your usual snack, try eating fruit. The concept here is to play with this thing. Find out what works for you. We are all different. Each and every one of us will find that our body, and therefore the rate at which we are losing pounds, reacts differently from everyone else's body. There are no "pat" answers. You have to educate yourself. You must determine how your body reacts to various stimuli.

There is one not so obvious technique that may or may not help you get off that plateau and back to losing pounds. And that is sleep. I mentioned earlier that a lack of sleep may cause a plateau. This may sound weird to you, but I found that getting an extra couple hours of sleep would sometimes help me get off that plateau. It is important that you get adequate amounts of sleep each night. If we get a good amount of sleep, we are able to maintain our physical activity level and, we generally feel better. And this is extremely important. If we feel good, our mental attitude will also be better. And it is this good mental attitude that is necessary to continue our efforts to change our lifestyle

Just consider what might happen if, for several nights, you got only half of your normal amount of sleep. Well, first of all, I'm sure you won't feel like taking your usual walk or playing some golf. And second, when we are tired, we usually head for the refrigerator or snack stand for some energy (food). And lastly, our attitude and enthusiasm suffer. We just don't feel like worrying about the quantity and quality of our food or activity for that matter. When we get tired, we also get complacent.

I had several experiences where my work load, drastically cut into my sleeping habits. And during these periods, my efforts to continue losing weight, at the desired rate, went completely haywire. On one occasion, I even went for a period of a week or so, gaining weight every single day.

And here's another little "tidbit" about sleep. Did you know that by controlling the temperature of your bedroom at night that you can influence the metabolic rate at which you burn calories? Sleeping at lower temperatures requires your body to burn more calories to stay warm.

And here's another little trick to prove this point. Weigh yourself immediately before you get into bed. And the next morning immediately weigh yourself when you get out of bed. Notice a difference? You could see as much as a three pound difference.

So watch for those plateaus and periods where your weight loss rate begins to diminish. Each time you realize this is occurring determine what it will take to get back to your desired weight loss rate. In other words, watch what's going on and, "BE IN CONTROL!"

And here's one last thought about how each additional change you make can help support your weight loss at the desired rate. And, of course, these additional changes can also get you moving off a plateau. I am going through this to emphasize the unlimited number of things to try and get off a plateau and start losing pounds at the rate you want. Let's say that at the outset of this effort, you have a dish of ice cream every night. And of course you have to have some chocolate or butterscotch syrup on the ice cream. Plain ice cream just doesn't cut it. And suddenly you stop losing weight at the desired rate. Well let's look at what you're eating. There are three things here. The first is the ice cream. The second is the quantity of the ice cream. And the third is the frequency of eating the ice cream (every night). Then there's three more issues concerning the syrup. First of course is the syrup itself. And secondly there's the quantity of the syrup. And lastly there's the frequency of the syrup. That is, how often you eat ice cream with the syrup as opposed to eating it without the syrup. So there are six things you can possibly change or modify. You could eat the combination every other night. Or you could have ice cream every night but only add syrup on weekends. Or you could have ice cream every other night and syrup only on Sunday night. Or you could have this favorite combination every night, but eat only half as much. Or you could substitute ice milk for the ice cream and use a sugar free-syrup. Or maybe you might consider some additional activity. On those nights where you don't have some evening ice cream, take a 15 minute walk. Try reducing the ice cream consumption. If that doesn't get you off the plateau, add the walk on the nights you don't have the ice cream. Play with this. Learn from it. Challenge yourself to do what is necessary to get back to the weight loss rate that you desire.

The point is that you have to determine what it will take to get off the plateau. And the lifestyle changes must be something you choose to accomplish that goal.

And here's something to think about. You have hit a plateau. And you decide to either stop eating toast with your breakfast for four consecutive mornings or take an additional 15 minute walk for four consecutive nights. Which do you think is the better choice to get off that plateau and start losing weight again? In a future chapter we are going to talk about calories. What do you think is better? You can reduce your calorie consumption by four pieces of bread or burn calories walking.

Here's a hint. If you weigh 180 pounds, you'll burn about 290 calories walking. And the four slices of bread constitute about 320 calories. And though the calories are about the same, you'll find that taking the walks will give you a much better chance of getting off that plateau. And here's a novel idea: do both.

And I'll give you one more idea, based on my experience. If you're trying to get off a plateau, try having a bowl of soup for a few meals. I found this to be very helpful in re-starting the weight loss.

AVOIDING PLATEAUS

Is it possible to avoid a plateau? Well, the answer is maybe. Or better stated, it may be possible to recognize that you are about to hit a plateau. I previously made the following statement. "So watch for those plateaus and periods where your weight loss rate begins to diminish." The key here is the phrase "periods where your weight loss rate begins to diminish." If you get really good at this technique, you may see an occasion where your weight loss rate begins to diminish. Let's say you are losing about one and one-half pounds per week. That equals about 6 pounds per month. That's a very good, safe and acceptable weight loss rate. But then all of a sudden you lose only one pound during an entire week and only a half pound the following week. I can just about guarantee that if you cannot attribute this change in your weight loss rate to some change in your lifestyle (for example eating more than usual or a decrease in your physical activities), then you are heading for a plateau. If you can attribute the weight loss rate decrease to some changes in your lifestyle, then you need to go back to the lifestyle that maintained your one and one-half pound per week weight loss rate. But if you didn't change anything and still your weight loss rate is decreasing, then make some additional changes in your lifestyle (eating and/or physical activity) to pick up the rate of weight loss. If you don't, you will experience a plateau. And you'll have to make the lifestyle changes anyway to get off the plateau. So if you recognize the weight loss rate decreasing, make the additional changes and avoid the plateau.

Chapter 14

ANNOTATING YOUR GRAPH

I previously mentioned the technique of placing a red dot on your graph on days you ate what you consider to be a larger than normal amount of food. I'm going to dig a bit deeper into this concept because it brings about an awareness of how eating and physical activity can affect your weight and desired weight loss rate. This technique is all about teaching yourself how to lose weight at your desired rate. I have talked about and will continue to talk about daily weighing and looking at your graph and determining how you're progressing. What you do today and tomorrow must be based upon your weight and where you stand in terms of your goal.

If you're inside your envelope and losing weight at your desired rate, then all you have to do is continue what you're now doing. But if you are having problems with a consistent weight loss rate, then to fix the problem you need to know why it's happening.

Take a look at the graph below. It's for a period of 25 days.

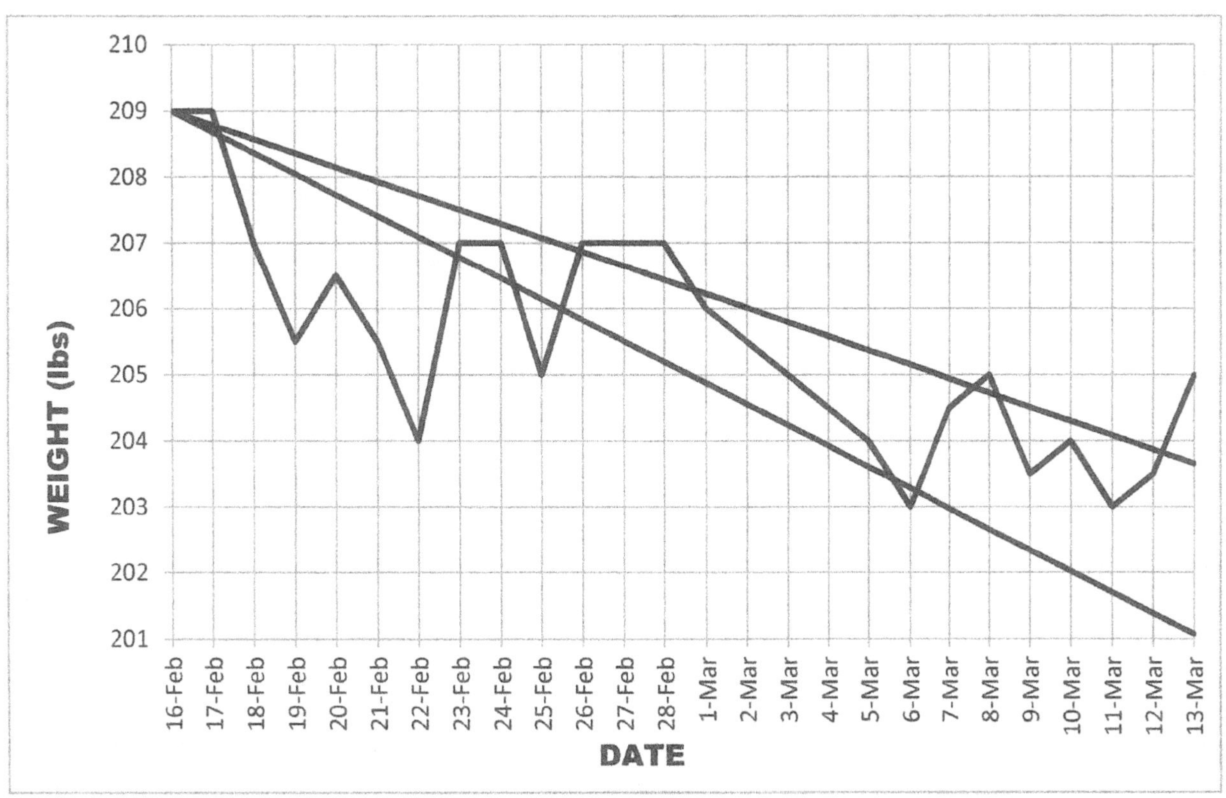

In looking at this graph, you see two periods of good consistent weight loss. You also see two periods that look like plateaus. And, you also see two periods of weight gain that led to those two plateaus. But what caused the weight gain of February 21st? And what happened on March 7th and 8th that caused the previous six or seven days of consistent weight loss to come to such a quick halt. And what caused the two pound increase on March 7th and 8th?

Well to answer these questions, look at the graph below.

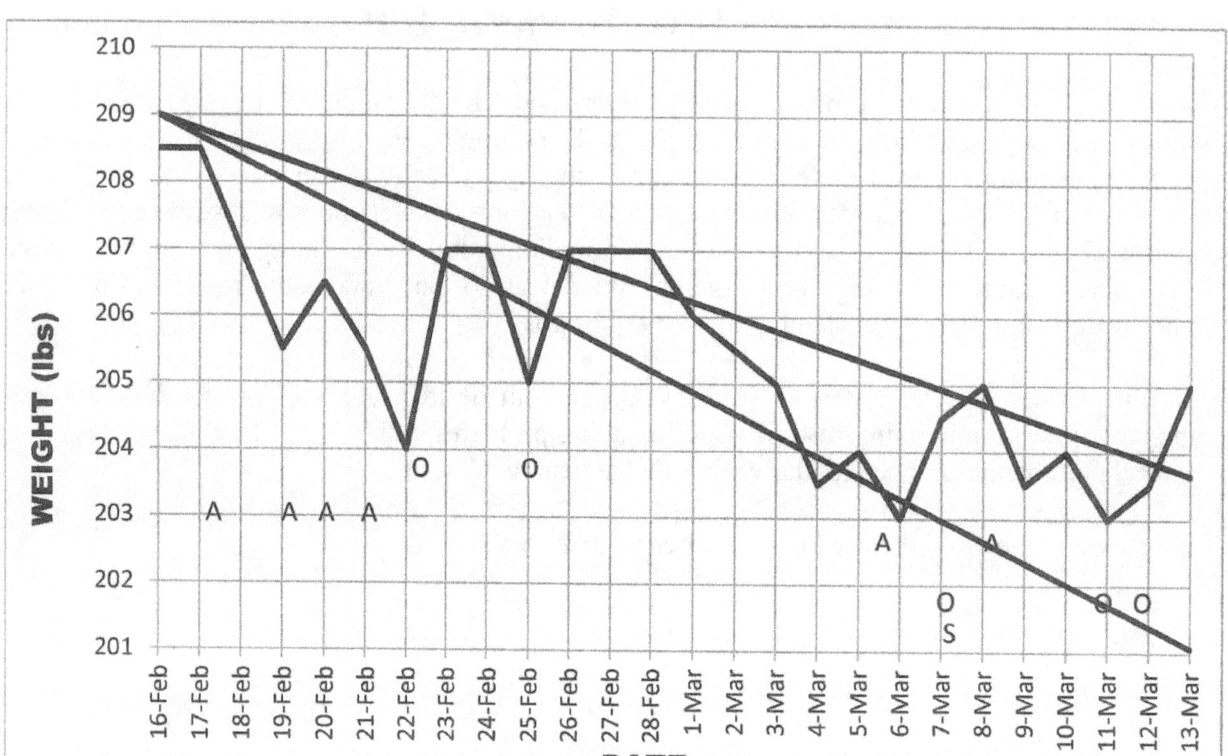

The letter "A" denotes days where a ½ mile walk was taken and the letter "O" denotes days where more than the normal amount of food was eaten. With these annotations, it is quite clear as to the reason for the variations in the rate at which weight was lost during this period. The only other modification made during this period was to stop all nighttime snacking with the exception of March 7th, when an evening piece of cake was eaten, denoted with the letter "S."

My recommendation is that you record this information in a notebook. That is, record days when you eat a bit more than normal, and record what activities you undertake each day. Then if something happens and you want to look at your graph and try and determine some reason for an abnormal weight variation, then put the dots, or letters on your graph and see if your lifestyle might give a clue about the abnormal weight variation.

You might even try some experimentation with this technique. Say for example your weight loss is going great and you always take a short evening walk. Stop taking the walk for three consecutive nights and change nothing else. Then see if your weight loss rate varies. I have never known this technique to not help solve problems and give insight as to the effects, both positive and negative, of lifestyle changes.

This is all part of the discovery process about your lifestyle, the changes to that lifestyle and the effects of those changes. This is how you learn about yourself and how you can make changes in your lifestyle to achieve your goal weight. This is the method to measure the positive effects of the lifestyle changes you make. And just as important, this is the technique you can use to see and determine the precise results of varying from the positive changes you have made. If you see, in looking at your graph, that you have suddenly stopped losing weight at your desired rate, this is the technique to help determine what may have caused this. It's all part of the discovery process. It's how you discover how your lifestyle affects your weight.

And for just a moment think about the E's and O's in term of calories. E's are days where calories burned probably exceeded calories consumed. If you burn more than you take in, you will lose weight. And O's are days where calories consumed probably exceeded calories burned through activities. If you take in more calories than you burn, you will gain weight. It's not rocket science.

And if you really want to get into the cause and effect thing, keep a log of what you eat every day, including meals and snacks. Also keep track of your activities. Then go back and relate your food intake and activities to your weight. I absolutely guarantee you will be astonished as what you can learn. There is a direct relationship between these factors and it will become obvious. And from this you can begin to educate yourself on what <u>not</u> to eat and what <u>to do</u> to ensure you continue your weight loss rate.

Chapter 15

CAUTION

I have talked about the dangers of trying to lose too much weight too fast. Primarily you've read about the physical dangers associated with a rapid weight loss. It is true that rapid weight loss can dangerously affect your health. But what I want to focus on here concerns the techniques often used for rapid weight loss. Primarily, a major reduction in caloric intake and at times a major increase in activity (caloric output), are the usual techniques utilized for rapid weight loss.

Let's assume that you undergo one of these rapid weight loss programs and through a drastic reduction in caloric intake, you lose 75 pounds. Instead of eating your usual 3000 calories a day, you get only 1500 calories a day. Even if you don't increase your level of physical activity, you will lose weight. If you do increase your level of activity, you'll lose the weight even faster. But, when you're finished with this program, and the doctor has released you (and I do hope you've been closely monitored by a doctor during this "diet"), you really haven't learned how to live properly. You've learned how to diet!

You can't live the way you were living while on the diet, that's for sure. You know of only two ways to live. The diet way; and the way you lived prior to the diet. And living that way is what caused you to need the diet in the first place. That's why so many people go on diets, only to regain the weight when they go off the diet. Rapid and major changes in food intake and levels of exercise are difficult to deal with physically and emotionally. These types of major changes, made rapidly, are practically impossible to maintain for long periods of time, especially the rest of your life. That's the problem with most diets. They don't prepare you for life after the diet.

In addition, as we get older our needs change as do our bodies. And if our diet doesn't take this into consideration, we begin to put on a few pounds here and there. And in most cases, this weight gain occurs over a long period of time. A businessman who works a somewhat sedentary job requires fewer calories than his 14 year old son, who is probably very active in sports. Many people realize this. This is the primary reason the health club business has done so well in recent years.

This technique of monitoring your weight every day and slowly modifying your living habits gives you the opportunity to self determine what level of activity and food intake you need. It also DOES NOT require you to stop eating the things you love. It does require an effort on your part to at least determine those food items that you know are contributing to your excessive weight and start reducing the amounts of these foods. But even the food reduction doesn't have to start right away. You could, if you like, just start increasing your level of activity. Watch your weight every day, and see what results you get from the increased activity. Remember that if you only slightly increase your activity level, it may take some time before you begin to see the results on your scale. Then, if you see no results, your body is telling you that you are taking in the exact number of calories that your are using. In other words, if you hadn't been undertaking that activity, you would have, in all probability, _gained_ some weight. If you see some weight loss from the increased activity, but want to lose weight at a somewhat faster rate, then try a small reduction in your food intake. Cut back a little on the size of your servings of food. Or maybe you could eat a light lunch two or three days each week. Again, watch your weight each day and try to relate your weight with each change in your living habits. You may decide to increase your level of activity. You may decide to stop snacking, or have a snack only every other night. Whatever works for you is great. But these little changes you make will each contribute to your weight. What you have to do is to watch your eating and activity habits, and relate the changes you have made to the weight changes you see on the scale each and every morning.

Here is the danger I mentioned before about over-challenging yourself. If you have set your goal too high, (in other words, if the two goal lines that make up the envelope on your graph are too steep) then you may have required yourself to make major changes in your life-style. If your desired weight loss rate is too high, then major changes in food intake are necessary, and maybe an excessive amount of activity is necessary. If this is the case, then your chances or maintaining this life-style after you've achieved your desire weight are rather slim.

Another way of looking at this is that if your two goal lines are too steep and you have to make major (and unpleasant) changes in your diet and activity, you are turning this journey into a conventional diet. There are two problems with this. First, it's an unhealthy approach. And second, you haven't prepared yourself for life after the diet. You surely aren't going to continue eating the small amounts of food and exercising at the level that you used to lose the weight. So, please don't over challenge yourself. This must be a slow process.

In addition, if you make a "whole bunch" of changes at one time, it is difficult to relate each change to your weight loss rate. And it is important to know how your body reacts to each modification you make. And minor modifications are much easier to endure. The whole key is to take it slow and learn from each experience. The number one benefit is that you begin to eat intelligently. Because you weigh yourself every morning, you tend to think about what you are going to eat.

We all know someone who has been on one of those diets where they go for a weekly "weigh-in." It is sometimes comical what they will do. They tend to starve themselves for the one or two days prior to the weigh-in. And the day after the weigh-in they figure, "well, I don't have to get weighed for seven days, so I'll have some desert." If you weigh yourself every day, and learn the results of your day to day eating habits (and activity habits) you will live each day differently. And you will find that if the changes you've made in your activity and eating habits are small changes, they are much easier to continue to the next day and the next day and the next day and so on. And eventually you will realize that you have taught yourself to live and eat intelligently. And, after some period of time, you will realize that you are eating very differently than before and are no longer aware of the changes you've made. By going slowly you maintain a level of comfort with the changes you have made in your lifestyle.

In talking to the people who have successfully lost weight using this technique, the one common factor is that they are amazed with their ability to maintain their new weight. Why is it so easy to maintain the new weight? It's simple. They changed there lifestyle VERY SLOWLY. These small changes became part of their life. And when they reached their new weight, they just continued to live in the way they had taught themselves. I know of one person, (the minister I mentioned previously) who reached his weight loss goal, and couldn't stop losing weight. He lost an additional 20 pounds beyond his goal. And when he reached the proper weight for his age and stature, he had to increase his food intake to maintain the physical activity (golf and evening walks) that he had come to love.

So remember the title of this chapter is CAUTION. There are two extremely important reasons for this CAUTION. First, it is UNHEALTHY to undergo a rapid weight loss. And this includes losing weight at a faster rate than the lower line of your envelope. In other words, it's dangerous to go below your lower goal line. Second, each modification you make must be small enough to easily maintain for the remainder of your life, if necessary. Why do I say "if necessary?" Well, that leads us to the next chapter. But I will only say here that certain activity and eating habits that you have learned may or may not be necessary for you to maintain your new weight. How will you determine which ones to maintain and which ones to stop? It is something you will have to find out for yourself. You may want to continue your physical activity because you have come to love it, as did the fellow above. Or you may want to decrease the amount of physical activity and maintain your current eating habits. It's entirely up to you. Really, I'm getting too much into the next chapter. So, I'll stop here and have you read the next chapter, titled MAINTENANCE.

Chapter 16

MAINTENANCE

Without a doubt there are many good aspects to this technique of losing weight. But the greatest aspect is that this is not a diet, "as we know it." It is a technique that helps you to teach yourself, through experience, how to slowly and effectively change your lifestyle (activity and eating) so you can achieve a more health lifestyle and weight. It is this lifestyle change that enables you to keep the weight off. That is why it is so important that you make changes in your activity and eating habits very slowly, and that the changes you make be taken in tiny steps, and that these changes are continued throughout your journey. If the changes you make are major, then chances are you won't continue these lifestyle changes after you've lost the weight. For example, let us consider two scenarios. John weighs 190 pounds, and has decided he wants to lose 20 pounds. Mary weighs 135 pounds, and yearns to weigh 115 pounds once again.

John has decided he will eat only broiled fish for the next two months, and will go to the fitness center every evening until he has lost the weight. And if he sticks to this routine, he will probably lose the 20 pounds.

Mary, on the other hand, is going to employ this technique of weighing herself every morning, plotting her weight on the graph, and slowly changing her lifestyle to safely lose the 20 pounds. She has started taking a 30 minute walk every other evening, has stopped snacking at the office during her mid-morning coffee break, has reduced her helpings of certain foods, and once or twice a week will have a light lunch.

Both John and Mary will, in all probability, both lose the 20 pounds they want to shed. John will probably lose his 20 pounds long before Mary. But one year from now, chances are very good that Mary will have kept the weight off. John, on the other hand will probably gain the 20 pounds back. That is of course assuming that John hasn't completely given up on a social life by continuing going to the fitness center every evening. And too, I doubt if John will continue eating broiled fish, especially if he doesn't like it.

The point is Mary changed her lifestyle. She initiated some activity. She changed her eating habits and will probably continue these habits after the 20 pounds are gone. What she did was not difficult. In fact, she would probably tell you it was quite enjoyable. John, on the other hand was, in all probability, miserable the whole time he was on his "diet." And as I stated before, it's a sure bet that John will return to the pre-diet lifestyle that caused him to gain the extra weight.

The fact is that Mary has changed her lifestyle to lose the weight and will, since the changes were made slowly, maintain the lifestyle she has created over the weeks or months. And by continuing this new lifestyle, she will keep the weight off.

However, we all slip back into bad habits once in a while. And the key is catching yourself in the early stages. To do this, I suggest you continue to weigh yourself every day, and plot your weight on a graph. You should not be amazed that your body weight will go through various seasonal cycles. We all tend to gain weight in the winter, due to a decrease in activity. By watching your weight (by means of the graph) you can catch a general tendency to gain weight long before it gets to the point where you realize your 10 pounds over your comfortable weight.

I suggest that once you reach the weight you desire, that you draw a red line on your graph about 5 or 10 pounds above that weight. In my case, this red line is drawn at 180 pounds. I have learned that above 180 pounds I don't feel good and I don't look good! Then by monitoring your weight each day, you can easily detect a tendency to gain weight by noticing that your weight is climbing toward that red line. If and when this happens, take appropriate action. If it is due to a seasonal lack of activity, determine what modifications you can make in your eating habits to compensate for this lack of activity. If, you realize that you haven't had time for your evening walk, either make time, or change your eating habits. The key is that the graph brings about an awareness of your body's reaction to the way you live. You may realize that you started gaining weight right after you joined the office bowling team. How can that be? Exercise is good for the body! True, but if you have a couple of beers, and a bag of chips while getting this "exercise," you can easily determine that your "losing ground" with this total activity. Remember - our lifestyle is made up of eating habits and activity habits. Each may (or must) compensate for a lack of one or an over-indulgence of the other.

One additional trick I use is based upon watching my weight with respect to the weight I know I should maintain. According to the medical charts, I should weigh about 180 pounds. So I watch my weight by determining each month how many days I am above 180 pounds, and how many days I am at or below 180 pounds. If the number of days above 180 is greater than the number of days at or below 180, then I have to figure out why and take appropriate action.

Now I know some of you are thinking to yourself, "Oh Brother! You mean I have to keep watching my weight for the rest of my life. I just wanted to lose some weight and then stop thinking about it." Okay. Use this graphical method to change your life-style and don't think about this chapter. Then when you've lost the weight, come back and read this chapter. What you will find, is that this technique is not a bother. It is a simple tool to help you maintain your newly developed lifestyle. Those of you who were upset at the thought of doing this forever are still thinking of this process as a diet. IT IS NOT A DIET !!!! You will, I hope, make many positive changes to your lifestyle. One of those changes is getting on the scale every morning. After you've lost the weight, you will, I hope, maintain these newly developed habits. And to help, you should maintain the habit of getting on the scale every morning and plot, or at least, be aware of your weight and those factors that contribute to it.

If you don't want to plot your weight on your graph, that's fine. Just weigh yourself every day and if you get say 2 or 3% above your desired weight, just make a concerted effort over the next two weeks to do what is necessary to get back to your desired weight. Use whatever technique works for you. But do weigh yourself every day so you can be aware of these trends. Don't wait until you can't get your shirt or blouse buttoned.

So, watch your weight. Be intelligent about how you treat your body. Take care of it, and it will reward you with many years of good health.

Chapter 17

THE REST OF THE STORY

I have shown you my monthly graphs for January through April. To allow you to view all aspects of my journey, here are the graphs for the months of May, June and July. As Paul Harvey said in his radio program, "Now you know the rest of the story."

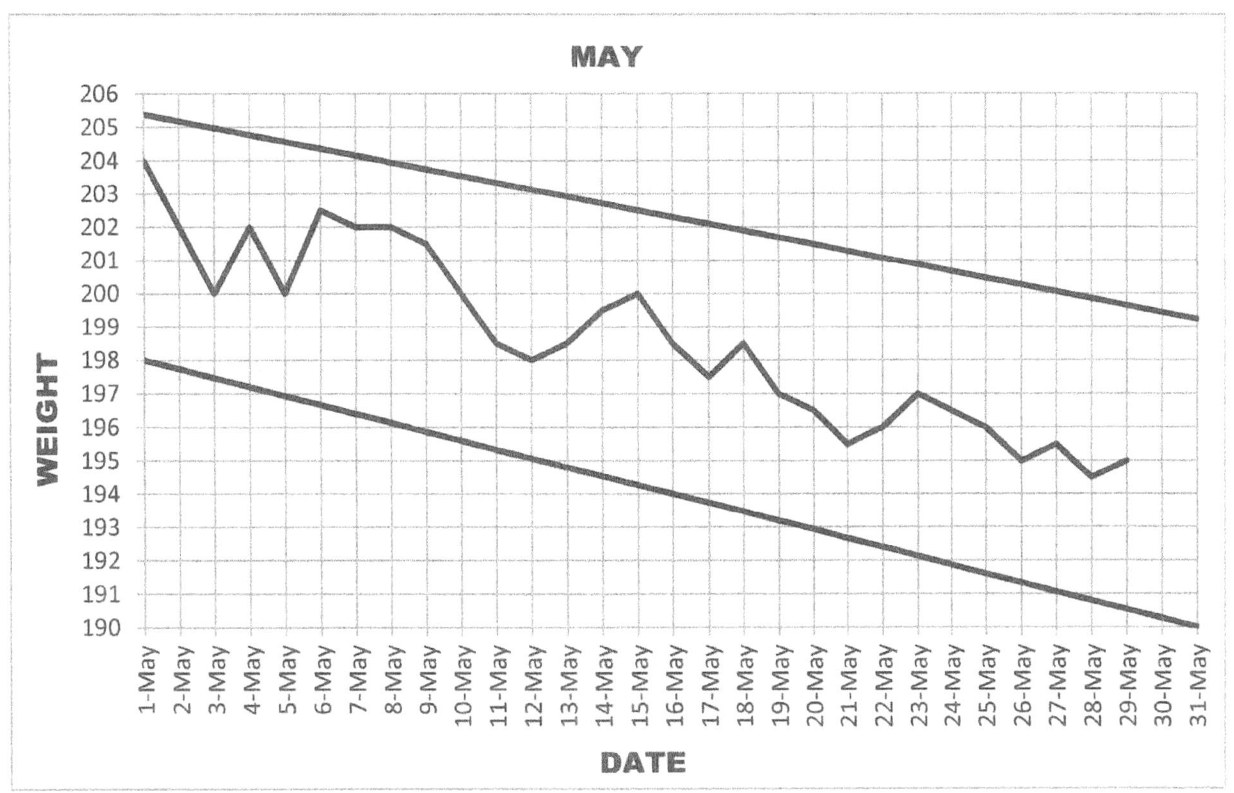

Nothing of any major consequence happened in May except you may notice that in the early days my weight was jumping around more than usual. Most of the time the variation of my weight was a half-pound to one pound from day to day. But here were five consecutive days where my weight varied between 1 ½ and 2 ½ pounds per day. I honestly do not know the reason for this. At this early stage I was not recording or making notes about my activity routines and eating habits from day to day. Had I been doing this, I guarantee that this type of weight variation could be tied to eating, physical activity, or some other issue. What could this "other issue" be? Well, it could very well be a physical change. There are many things that can happen to you that would cause your weight to vary more than normal from day to day. For example, what if you got a 24 hour virus? If you didn't eat much on a given day due to the flu, you might see a large loss the next day. If you have a severe cold and are drinking lots of fluids for a couple of days, your weight may show abnormal gains for those couple of days. That is the beauty of weighing yourself every day. The vast majority of the time you can relate your daily weight to something.

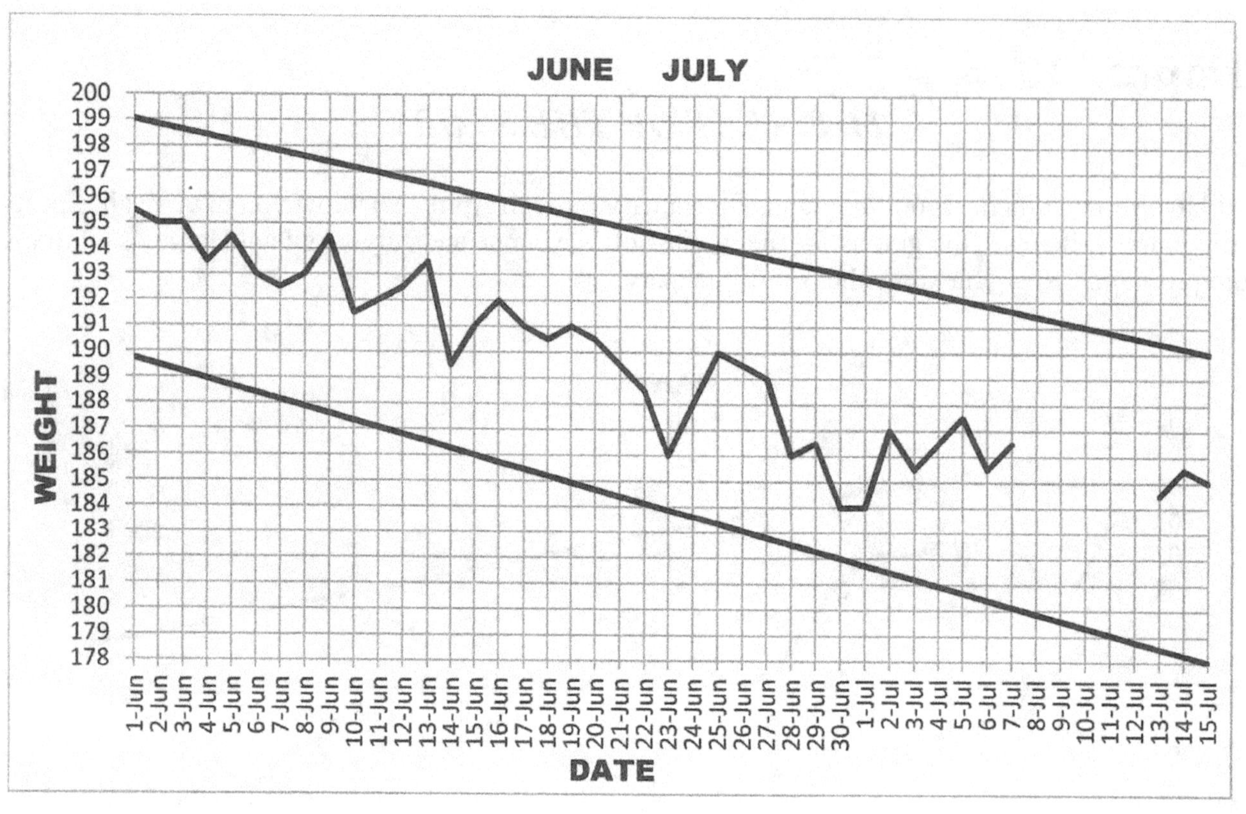

And here's the graph for June and the first half of July. Recall that my goal date was July 15th. So that's where my chart stops. There are a couple of things to notice here. First, take a look at the period from June 7th to June 14th. This stair step type of activity is quite common. You will find it in many of my graphs and I'm sure it will occur on your graphs. It is quite normal to go a day or two where you might gain a half pound or maybe a full pound. When this happens, you must react with some action to counteract this trend. For example, on June 11th and June 12th I gained a half pound each day. The on June 13th I gained a full pound. Had I <u>not</u> noticed this and taken some action to counter this trend, it may have continued to where I was gaining weight or stopped losing. You may also realize that this stair step period is almost like a plateau. If you look at June 7th, my weight was 192 ½ pounds. On June 16th, my weight was 192 pounds. That means I lost only ½ pound in 9 days. I made some changes in my lifestyle to get off the plateau. And look what happened during the period from June 17th to June 23rd. I lost 8 pounds in that 7 day period. You will find this happens quite often. You hit a plateau or a period where you don't lose much weight. You make some lifestyle changes and, all of a sudden, you lose 5, 6, or 7 pounds over a period of a week or so. You will find that your pounds will disappear in spurts.

Here's one last comment. Notice that on July 1st, my weight was 184 pounds and over the next six days it went up to 186 and stayed there. Well, it was another plateau. Unfortunately, I had a week long business trip (which is why there was no weight for July 8th through the 12th). During this trip, I was unable to continue my activities and, as I said before, it is quite difficult to monitor your eating when traveling. This trip was such that I had very limited flexibility in my choices of food. I worked long hours and got less than the ideal amount of sleep. Once the trip was over, I had only three days to try and create some type of downward trend. Given what had taken place from July 2nd through the 12th, there wasn't much of a chance to get that downward trend started.

All in all, I was extremely pleased with the result of my attempt to change my lifestyle. I had gone from about 250 pounds to 185 pounds in 9 ½ months. And I hadn't weighed 185 pounds since my early high school days. Upon returning from my mid July vacation, I created some additional charts, and eventually got down to 175 pounds; three pounds below my recommended weight. I lost 75 pounds in less than one year.

I suspect that right now you are thinking to yourself that one year is a long time to be on this journey. My comment is this. First, it took a lot longer to gain those 75 pounds. I suspect it probably took fifteen years for me to go from 175 to 250 pounds. And actually, I had weighed as much as 270 in the year prior to "my Journey." And I didn't gain that weight "pigging out" on one or two specific foods. I developed some very bad eating habits over those years. And I had drifted into a very sedentary lifestyle. Of course as a young boy, playing baseball wasn't exercise. It was fun. And there's another key to the success of this process. During this journey, I didn't exercise. I took walks and played golf and enjoyed it, just as I did when I was young and weighed 185.

This was a most pleasant and rewarding experience. It never felt like it was a chore. It was an exciting time for me because I was in control. I was so thrilled about what I was learning about myself and how I was able to actually control the rate at which I lost weight. Before, my weight controlled me. Now I was in control. I was excited about the new me and the fact that I was doing this on my own. I never really believed I would ever be able to lose this kind of weight. Why? Because I didn't like all the foods that I believed you must eat to lose weight.

Be honest with yourself. Are you of the opinion that to lose weight you must eat salads? Don't you think that if you're like me and love peanut butter, that you must "give it up." You don't have to give up the things you love. Do you remember that I mentioned french fries a couple of times in previous chapters? Well, I'll use the french fries to summarize this entire journey. Yes, french fries can be bad for you. But they are bad for you only if you eat them frequently and in large quantities. But I will say this. I eat them much less frequently. And sometimes, even though they come with my steak, I just don't eat them. I love to leave them on the plate and prove to myself that I don't want them.   I don't want the pleasure of eating those delicious french fires at the expense of my physical well-being. And if I get a burger with my fries, I may not eat the bun that comes with it. Or maybe I'll eat just the lower bun and leave the top half – I don't need those carbs.

You see, I'm in control!

And about those salads. You have to eat salads to lose weight. Right? Guess what. I hate salads and I have never in my entire life eaten a salad and I never will. I don't like them and I will not eat them – period.

Chapter 18

ALL THE OTHER DIETS

Let's talk a bit about all the other diets out there. Now I will agree that they all can work for some people. Many people have in fact lost weight on the various diets. But have you ever wondered why there are so many successful diets? There are countless numbers of people who will tell you, "I've tried all kinds of diets, and this particular one or that particular one was the first one that worked for me." Why do they all seem to work? Why is one diet where you eat lots of grapefruit successful, where another diet tells you to avoid this type of fruit because of the sugar? And then you find that that second diet was also successful for many people. If the sugar is so detrimental, why did the person lose weight? What do you think is the one common factor in every diet that's out there? If you buy all the books on the various diets, you will not find the one common issue. Well then, what is it? It's the fact that the people on these diets are probably for the first time, paying attention to the food they eat. They, because they are in a mental state of "I'm on a diet," are therefore paying attention to what they are eating and consume less, or completely stop eating the many "bad" foods they crave. But what happens when they go "off" the diet? Are they going to eat grapefruit the rest of their life, or continue to buy the special meals?

You will find many diets that have you eating very special low calorie and low fat foods. Many times it is so special that you have to purchase the food from them or buy their brand. The problem is not that you won't lose weight. You could very well lose weight. Many people are successful on these diets. But without some activity, you could also lose muscle (which by the way weighs more than fat). We'll talk more about burning calories in just a bit. Secondly, once the weight is gone, are you going to purchase their food for the rest of your life? Probably not. You have not therefore, changed your living habits in a way you can live for the rest of your life. So, you gain the weight back. Then lose it again. Then gain it back again and hopefully lose it again. I say hopefully, because each time you gain weight back it seems to be a little more difficult to get rid if it the next time. And let's face it, this roller coaster ride is heart wrenching and demoralizing. And recent studies are also beginning to suspect this type of dieting is unhealthy in that it has all kinds of detrimental and negative effects.

And what happens if you're traveling. Maybe you can't eat those special meals you have been buying and heating in the microwave. And if you go out for dinner, what then? Maybe the special food you have been eating isn't on the menu. Or, your favorite aunt didn't know you can only eat special types of food. She prepared a beautiful delicious and probably nutritious meal. But since none of your special foods are on the table what do you do now? You just have to learn to eat more selective and limit the quantities of those foods that are not ideal. And guess what! That is precisely what this process allows you to teach yourself. Through trial and error and watching your daily weight, you will teach yourself how to eat more intelligently and achieve and maintain a healthy weight.

In examining the various diets I have another question that has to be answered. Why do some of these diets work for some people and don't work for others.   Let's take a look at Mary. Mary has been overweight for many years. She would love to slim down a bit, but well, she was just never able to succeed in losing weight. Mary tried diet A and diet B. She didn't lose any weight. But when she went on Diet C, she lost weight. Sue couldn't lose weight on Diet A and Diet B. But she lost twenty five pounds on diet C. Why is this? I believe there are two issues. And the success of any effort to lose weight depends on these issues in varying degrees. Let's take a look at Mary's diets. The first issue is commitment and attitude. Is it possible that Mary's commitment and attitude on diets A and B wasn't very strong? But when Mary heard her best friend talking about her (Mary's) dress size, she made a more firm commitment and she started diet C and lost weight. And now she says that diet C is so much better than the other two. It wasn't the diet. It may have been her commitment or lack of commitment that resulted in the success or failure of the diets. The second issue is comfort. Is it also possible that diets A and B were based on foods that Mary just doesn't like? She may have tried to cultivate a taste for salads, but just doesn't like the leafy stuff. Diet C may have allowed her to eat more of the food types that she likes. So, she was much more comfortable with her lifestyle while on diet C. But what are the chances that Mary will keep the weight off? Well the answer to that one is totally dependent upon whether Mary's diet (diet C) prepared her for a lifestyle after the diet. Chances are it didn't. Chances are she will declare the diet "over," and return to her pre-diet lifestyle.

And in addition, many of these diets place too much emphasis on the food side of the issue. In a later chapter we will talk about the balance of calories coming in (foods consumed) and calories going out (activity). Inventing ways to burn calories is also a very important factor in losing weight, and maintaining both a healthy weight and a healthy body, which includes good muscle tone, good lung capacity, a healthy heart, healthy blood vessels, and all the other benefits that come from some levels of activity.

Now I will grant that some diets also address exercise. Oh, how I hate that word. When you read that last sentence and came upon the word exercise, didn't you conjure up images of some poor person on a treadmill in a health club sweating like crazy and wishing like you-know-what that he or she were somewhere else? But again most of these diets don't address the exercise as a factor of lifestyle change. They address it as a temporary way of burning calories at a high rate. They want you to be successful at losing weight on their diet. So they have you sweating at the gym or doing "sit-up crunches" on your bedroom floor. They are trying to assure you burn more calories than you take in. And this is great. That's precisely what you need to do. But the approach is all wrong. They are simply trying to make your "diet" (their diet) successful. And it may very well work and you will lose weight. And you will applaud this particular diet and tell all your friends about how successful it was and then they will run out and buy that book or join that plan or start buying those particular meals. But we have two problems. First, it was probably your commitment that was the primary reason the diet worked for you. And maybe your friend doesn't have the same commitment. So they start on the diet and it's a complete failure. It wasn't the diet that was the primary reason you were successful and they weren't. It was the commitment. The second problem is will you keep the weight off. Chances are you won't. Why? Well, you learned how to "diet.' You didn't learn how to change your lifestyle for the long term.

And you know there is a difference between activity and exercise. You may not agree with me, but I think there is a major difference in the image each word creates. For example, let's talk about walking. Taking a 30 minute walk with your dog in the evening is an activity. Spending 30 minutes on a treadmill going nowhere is exercise. And which is more enjoyable?

Chapter 19

CALORIES

Ok. So we've talked about the graph and you have hopefully created yours. We've talked about the attitude and the commitment and hopefully you have addressed the issues within yourself and have made a commitment to undertake this journey. The attitude? Well, I hope you have worked on that as well and have taken the attitude that after all these years it is time to do something, and you are going to do it. And, we've talked about some of the pitfalls and problems you will encounter along the way. But we haven't talked a great deal about some of the things that you can do that will help. We've touched on a few, but only in passing. There are things you can do to get started; to reduce the length of your "start" period. There are things you can do to help get off a plateau, or at least shorten the length of time you're on that plateau. You must also remember to not lose weight too fast. You don't want to lose weight faster than the lower envelope line. So, there are some things to slow down your weight loss. Now you might be thinking to yourself. There's not much chance of that happening. Or, maybe your thinking, boy would I love to have that problem. Well it can happen, and as I said many times, the results can be catastrophic. The key is to take it slow. Remember, this isn't a diet! It is a very slow methodical way of changing the way you live. And those changes are all geared toward a better lifestyle. You're going to take your current lifestyle and gradually modify it to lose weight at a very slow and healthy pace and in the end, create a lifestyle that will provide you with many years of good health.

And it's important you understand another reason for taking it slow and not losing the weight too fast. If you make drastic changes in your eating habits or undertake a strict and vigorous exercise regiment or do both, you may lose the weight very quickly. But I guarantee you will gain it back. You have not formulated a new lifestyle. You have not slowly evolved into a new and improved lifestyle. You have in essence gone on a diet and strenuous exercise routine. And these techniques do not work for the long haul. You've gone too fast. It's not smart and it's certainly not healthy to lose weight this way. Don't do it. Stay inside your envelope!

First of all, it should come as no surprise to learn that losing weight is all about what you eat and what you do. The next three chapters are going to address the various aspects of this topic. We will talk about calories in this chapter.   And we'll talk about food content, nutrition, meals, snacking, and various ideas about eating and burning calories in the next chapters.

Losing weight is all about the numbers. And I'm not talking about the number of pounds to be lost or the number of pounds to be lost per month (rate). The numbers I'll be talking about concern calories. I've touched on this earlier, but since it is very important that you fully understand this concept, I will delve into it a bit more. And don't worry about having to buy a special calculator and start counting calories. That is not what this is about. This is not about counting calories so that you never consume more than 1300 calories per day or some other magic number. That type of dieting doesn't work for the long run. It's not about calorie counting, but developing smart eating habits. This is not about the 250 calories in that caramel nugget candy bar that we all love. But you must understand that calories being burned through activity versus calories eaten results in losing weight, or gaining weight, or maintaining your current weight. If you have gained weight in recent years, it is simply because you're taking in more calories than you're burning. And those extra calories are stored in the body as fat. And as I have stated before, as we age, we tend to be less active, we lose muscle-mass and our metabolism changes. Thus if we continue to eat like we did at a younger age, and because we are getting older, are burning fewer calories, then it is a simple fact that we may gain weight. For some, this never happens. Their metabolism is such that they stay thin their entire life.

Everything you do consumes calories. As I stated in a previous chapter, you burn calories just sleeping.   If you consume 3000 calories in one day and through your daily activities you burn only 2150 calories, you will gain weight. It's that simple. If on the other hand you consume 2500 calories per day and you burn 3000 calories per day, you will lose weight. If the numbers are approximately the same, you will maintain your current weight. This process is not rocket science. It is simply a question of what we eat (quality and quantity), and how much we burn through activity.   And here I go again. The quantity is extremely important. We eat too much!

Let's say that a helping of Lasagna contains 400 calories. If you have been eating two helpings and now cut back to one helping, you have just saved 400 calories. Studies have shown the average person consumes about 2700 calories per day. And for the person of average height and weight, they should consume 2000 calories per day. That's a 26% reduction. If you have been consuming 2700 calories per day and you pass on the second helping of lasagna, you just (for the day) reduced your caloric consumption by about 15%. How far do you think you would have to walk (in the park or on the treadmill) to burn 400 calories?   A person weighing 130 pounds would have to walk for over 2 hours and 45 minutes. And a 200 pound person would have to walk for 2 hours to burn those 400 calories. And if you don't walk for two hours to burn off those calories, guess where the calories get stored?

Even our young children are becoming more obese. Why? Well, it doesn't take a brilliant scientist to figure this one out either. TV, video games, the internet, lack of funds resulting in the removal of physical education programs in our schools all contribute to the problem.   The quality of the food our children are eating is much, much worse than twenty or thirty years ago. The amount of sugar consumed is vastly greater than what it was in the 19th century. And though it is true that the increasingly sedentary lifestyle of many children is a contributor, the primary culprit to this problem is the amount of food our children consume and the quality of that food. The "fast food" craze is taking a toll on our younger generation.

And it is not just the "fast" food craze that has taken a toll on our lifestyle. For example, take a walk down two aisles in your local grocery. First, look at the number of available cereals that are loaded with honey, and sugar coatings. We have taken a very good source of fiber and loaded it with fat and sugar to make it taste better and get our children to want that food and to want that taste. And look at the number of cookies that again have sugar coatings and contain chocolate. Are these items all that bad? Well, not really. But a bowl of that sugar coated or honey laden cereal every morning can be disastrous if the child also has a very sedentary lifestyle. And how many of you see children put two or three teaspoons of additional sugar on their cereal. And a chocolate chip cookie is not inherently bad. But having six of these cookies after a complete and filling lunch can be catastrophic.

And it is not affecting just the young generation. Many adults are guilty of succumbing to these types of foods as well. And once again, it is not just the food. There is a second side to this equation. What is the activity lifestyle? High calorie foods can be consumed by people with very active lifestyles without negative consequences. So what it comes down to is this. To avoid gaining weight, you need to burn all of the calories you take in. And to lose weight, you need to burn more calories than you take in.

And here is a very important key to this whole process. You have an unlimited number of ways you can achieve the burning of more calories than you take in. Your choices are absolutely unlimited. And you don't have to make all of these decisions at the beginning of your journey. In fact you don't want to make all the decisions at the beginning. As I stated before, this is a slow methodical process of change. Each day or each week or each month you can decide to do a little bit more toward better health. And how much should you do? Well, that depends totally on your graph and how you are doing relative to your goal. You can decide to reduce your caloric intake a bit or initiate some activity, or do both. And notice I said activity. I purposely did not say exercise. The word exercise has that "link" to the dieting world. Though they are the same thing, the word exercise makes you think that the activity is not the normal way of spending an afternoon. Do you think that Chris Evert or John McEnroe ever said to someone, "Well I have to go exercise," as they went on the tennis court to play a match? It's not "exercise" to them. It's their way of life. So like the word diet, don't use the word exercise.   If someone notices you have slimmed down and they ask what exercises you are doing, tell them you're not exercising; just taking a walk several nights each week or describe whatever you are doing. Maybe you tell them, "I've been riding my bike." Oh they reply, "Exercising on your bike, eh?" And you answer, "No, I'm taking a leisure tour of my neighborhood on my bike, and I love it." You see, it's all about the attitude. Okay. I'll quit harping about "exercise."

Now there are various methods you can utilize to achieve caloric imbalance; expending more than you take in. If you decide you are going to lose weight but decide not to reduce the quantity of food you consume and also decide not to address the quality of that food, then you better buy a Winnebago motor home and park it in the health club parking lot. Why? Well, if you're not going to reduce the number of calories you're taking in, then you have to increase the number of calories you burn. On the other hand, if you decide that you are not going to increase your activity, but just lose the weight by cutting back on what you eat, then I suggest you still buy the motor home. Just move it from the health club parking lot to the parking lot at the local hospital emergency room. And though admittance to the hospital could be the result of physical problems (over exertion comes to mind), it cold also result from depression. This is an absolutely miserable way to lose weight. And, it is not necessary. And, it is not smart! And thirdly, you're not modifying your lifestyle for the long haul.

You could try the "apple" diet. Or you could try the "north mountain" diet. Or you could try "Dr. So-and-so's" diet. Or you might try the "carb-busters" diet or the "pounds viewers" diet. All of these diets can work for you as they do for others because they bring about an awareness of what you are eating. Of course, in some cases, they direct what you are eating. And they get rich at your expense. You don't have to make someone else rich to lose weight! The difference between these "diets" and the journey you are undertaking is that <u>you</u> are going to decide what you will eat. And <u>you</u> will decide how much of these items you will eat and what activity you are going to undertake. And <u>you</u> will make all of your decisions based upon the results of your previous decisions. In other words, how are you doing? Are you staying in your envelope? Are you losing weight at a rate that is slightly less than the rate of your upper line? In other words, are you getting close to your upper goal line? If so, it's time to either cut some calories (quality or quantity) or slightly increase your level of activity to stay below the upper goal line and above the lower goal line. You are going to guide yourself and make many decisions to do what it takes to lose weight at the rate you have committed to. In other words you are going to change your lifestyle to stay inside your envelope.

Okay. So let's concentrate on the topic of this chapter. The idea is to burn more calories than you consume. We all know that activity is the way you burn calories. But what about the calories in the food we consume. How do we intelligently watch our calorie consumption? What is the "bad" source of calories? Is it fat? Is it sugar? Is it Carbohydrates? And are there good calories? The answer to the first question is practically everything we eat contains calories. And the answer to the remaining questions is, yes.   Fat, sugar, and carbohydrates are all a source of calories. And all calories are good. The calorie is a technical term that defines a unit of energy. So, we have to have calories to live. The calorie is our body's source of fuel. Have you ever had the situation with an older car where your car engine won't start and the mechanic tells you that you "pumped" the gas peddle too much and flooded the engine? If you put too much fuel into an engine it will not run. If you put too much fuel into us, we will stall (get fat) and also cease to run (live).

So, we want to burn more calories than we take in. The difference between these two numbers defines your rate of weight loss or the slope of the upper line of your envelope. To accomplish this you have to be creative in your eating and your activities. There are no steadfast rules. Well, actually, that's not true. There are two rules. Your rate of weight loss must be reasonable and you must stay inside your envelope. That's it. Those are all the rules. In other words, there are no rules about how you do that. Let's start with the eating side of things. We've already determined that to lose weight you need to burn more calories than you consume. There are other elements of food that you have to consider as well. There's fiber. And there's cholesterol. Then there's fat. And there's sugar.   There's salt. And there are carbohydrates. And you need some of each of these things. You just have to watch the quantity of each. And some have more influence on your weight than others.

Three of these items, sugar, fat and carbohydrates are very closely tied to calories. Sugar is a high calorie item and therefore, is an energy food. A marathon runner requires a lot of energy. He or she will expend a massive amount of calories in running the marathon.   Does that mean that the marathon runner can eat 25 candy bars before a race? Candy bars are loaded with sugar. Sugar is energy and the runner needs energy. Well, those candy bars also contain fat. And the fat in those 25 candy bars is not good. So what does the marathon runner do? He eats a large amount of pasta. Pasta contains large amounts of carbohydrates. And carbohydrates turn to sugar when he or she digests the pasta. So the runner gets his or her energy (calories) and with very little fat. This technique is quite common and is called carbo-loading. In fact, I know of one marathon that has a dinner-party the night before the race and they serve vast amounts of pasta to the participants. So, the first idea is to limit the amount of sugar you take in. And in a like manner, you must watch your carbohydrates.

Now I know that there are some products that are sugar free, and carbohydrate free, and fat free. The problem is many of these are also taste free. In fact, the box they came in probably tastes better than the food. But there are some very good tasting foods out there that are sugar free. But, be very careful. A sugar free food could be loaded with carbohydrates and loaded with fat. In a like manner, many foods are advertised as fat free and contain enormous amounts of sugar. For several years, the food industry was concentrating on "fat free." That was the buzz word, and people were buying these items and could not understand why they weren't losing weight. The answer is that they were loaded with sugar. And sugar is a high calorie item. And if the person eating this food was not expending sufficient calories through their daily activity, they would not lose weight. The point is that you have to be aware of all food content. And don't allow the advertising world to move your attention away from all the important elements of the food you eat. For example, there is a potato chip that is advertised as 25% less fat. That's good. Right? Well, yes, that's good. It also contains no cholesterol and no sugar. But just a handful of chips contain 18 grams of carbohydrates. And is that bad? Well, as I've said before no food is totally bad. Some foods have larger amounts of some elements that we need to limit. But food is not inherently bad. There is one low carb diet that says you should limit you total daily intake to 20 grams of carbohydrates. And those low fat potato chips (just about a dozen chips) constitute 90% of the daily allowed intake of carbohydrates allowed on that diet.

A typical example of this dilemma is peanut butter. I choose this particular food item because I absolutely love the stuff. Peanuts are very high in protein and protein builds muscle. That's good. But peanut butter is loaded with fat, and some brands are very high in sugar. And that can be bad, depending on how much you consume. Well, the answer is not necessarily to give up peanut butter, but select one that contains less sugar. There are also places where you can buy natural peanut butter that contains very little sugar and fat. I have seen some grocery stores that make it for you right there in the store and add no sugar. And what about the fat, you ask? Well, the fat is not necessarily the problem. The problem, in my opinion, is the sugar. We'll talk more about the fat a bit later.

Sugar free colas and sugar free gum are also items that can help to reduce your calorie input. And as you can well imagine there are countless foods out there that are inherently very low in sugar. However, if you're like me, these low sugar food items are not the foods I like. But again, you don't have to give up the high sugar foods. Just eat less of these items when you decide to have some. And eat them less frequently.

I mention fruits throughout this book. Apples, oranges, bananas, pears are all good foods. And yes there are some diets that will tell you to avoid some of these because they are loaded with carbohydrates and natural sugars. But again, those diets are taking extreme positions. Let's talk about the carbohydrate position. It is true that oranges and orange juice have high amounts of carbs. But this journey you are undertaking is not a carb free diet. And fruits also contain other important nutrients. Think of it this way. You're not on a fat free diet and you're not on a carb free diet. You're looking for a healthier list of foods to eat. Consider this situation. It's 7:45 PM and you're feeling a bit hungry. You have decided you're not going to eat anything after 8:00 PM. Breakfast isn't until 6:00 AM. That means this snack must "hold you over" for 10 hours. You have two choices. You can have about a dozen crackers with peanut butter on them, or you can have an orange. They both contain sugar. They both contain carbs. The peanut butter is high in protein. The orange is high in vitamin C. Which do you think is better for you? Or you could be inventive and have some apple with just a touch of peanut butter on the slices of apple. That way, you can avoid the crackers, which are loaded with carbs, and if the peanut butter is low in sugar you can still fulfill your love of that food item. And guess what? Some people will tell you it is delicious!

I will share one bit of info with you. As I mentioned before, limiting carbohydrates is a good method of avoiding hunger. It may be that the peanut butter snack will hold you over, whereas the orange may leave you hungry again at 11:30 PM. What should you eat? What's the answer? I don't have an answer. And that's the beauty of this process. You have to experiment and find out what works for you, with the primary goal to stay inside your envelope.

Do you remember the 250 calorie candy bar I mentioned earlier? I stated that this is not about the 250 calories in the caramel nugget candy bar we all love. What I want you to understand is that you don't need to count calories. I don't care how many calories are in that candy bar. I don't need to know how many calories it contains. All I need to know is that it is high in calories and loaded with sugar, fat, and carbohydrates and I don't need any excesses of these items. You can go out and find a fat free food only to discover it is loaded with sugar. And that may be even more dangerous than the fat. Remember, we consume ten times more sugar than our grandparents. I need to make intelligent choices when it comes to selecting those items I will eat. But I love that candy bar! Okay. Then have just a half or a third and save the rest for tomorrow night. If you have been eating that candy bar every night and now just have ½ every night, you just reduced your calorie intake by 50%.

And you might even think to yourself … I just finished riding my bike five miles or I just walked two miles. And now I'm going to totally undo it all by eating a 250 calorie candy bar? Not on your life! You see, I'm in control!

You want proof of all of this? Well, In February of 2009, an Associated Press article reported on a study in the New England Journal of Medicine. The results stated that the kind of diet, low-fat, low-carb or high protein, didn't matter. All that really mattered was cutting calories. The key was to limit the calories consumed (eating) and burn off more calories with exercise (ugh – there's that word again). The study placed overweight adults on one of four different diets that were similar to existing popular diets. They were all asked to reduce the number of calories taken in by a specific amount (which means they had to count calories – oh what fun that is) and to exercise (Yuck! There it is again) for at least 90 minutes per week. The four diets contained healthy fats, whole grains, fruits and vegetables and were low in cholesterol. No one diet resulted in more weight loss than any other diet and weight reduction was the same in all groups. Didn't I say in an earlier chapter that all diets can work? It's not the diet, but the attitude and commitment and whether it was a diet that the dieter could endure. But here's the "kicker." People lost an average of 13 pounds in six months. However, all groups saw their weight increase after a year. And, after two years, the participants lost an average of nine pounds. Let's see, if they lost 13 pounds in the first six months, and lost only a total of nine pounds after 24 months, then the way I calculate it, in the last 18 months, they gained 4 pounds. I don't know about you, but I wouldn't want to go on any of those diets. And, all groups saw their weight increase after a year! The diets didn't teach anybody anything about an improved lifestyle!

The report stated that fifteen percent of the dieters did achieve a weight loss of ten percent or more of their starting weight. I would love to know how all the participants will do in the coming years. In other words, how many will gain the weight back and how many can keep it off for ten years?

The report stated that dieters who got regular counseling saw better results. Let's think about that for a minute. What do you think the counseling consisted of? Probably each participant talked with a counselor, or possibly a nutritionist, about their weight loss thus far, what they were eating and what exercise (ugh) they were performing. And when <u>you</u> sit down and look at <u>your</u> graph and analyze it in terms of what activity <u>you</u> are undertaking and think about how <u>you</u> can get back in your envelope (if you're outside of it) or off that plateau, just what do you think is taking place. You are conducting your own counseling session. You are teaching yourself. You're leading yourself to a better lifestyle. You don't need an expensive counselor to tell you what is working for you. You are going to teach yourself what works.

The report also said that those who attended most counseling sessions shed more pounds than those who did not attend the counseling sessions. What do you think is the reason for this improved success? Well, I think the more frequent counseling sessions brought about a greater awareness of the dieters progress and resulted in improved weight loss. And don't you think that by weighing yourself every morning and putting that weight on your graph and looking at that graph that you aren't conducting a personal counseling session every single day? And don't you think that increased (daily) awareness will result in a better chance of achieving the final desired weight?

The lead researcher stated, "They just need to focus on how much they're eating." He also stated that the trick is finding a healthy diet that is tasty and that people will stick with over time. Gee, I couldn't have said it better!

And I'll make one more comment from a personal point of view. Did you catch the foods that were eaten on the research study diets? The foods were healthy fats, whole grains, fruits and vegetables and were low in cholesterol. I don't know about you but if I had to eat that way for two years, I'd never make it. And that is the problem with most all diets. They often require you to eat foods that do not make the diet an enjoyable experience. That reduces the chances of success. And if the diet is successfully concluded and you go back to the lifestyle that you know (and the one that led to your overweight condition where the number of calories consumed was greater than those burned through activity) you will regain the weight.

Folks, you don't have to give up the things you love. If they are high in fat, sugar, carbs etc., you just have to eat less of these tasty items. And that will reduce your daily calorie intake. In fact, there may very well come a day when you won't want that tasty item. And you have to increase your level of activity to burn off more calories than you consume. And how about the "stick with it over time" issue. Well, what the researcher was getting at is that for a diet to successfully change your life, you must "stick with it over time." Otherwise, you'll gain the weight back. But these diets don't teach you that. They teach you how to diet! That's the beauty of this journey. You will modify your eating habits and activity habits slowly and change your lifestyle to one that you like and will continue.

I want to go back to one sentence in the previous paragraph. The report stated that what the researcher was getting at is that for a diet to successfully change your life, you must "stick with it over time." Let me ask you a question. What "diet" do you think the researcher was talking about? Was he or she talking about the research project, that is, the "diet" the participants just completed? Or was the researcher talking about the quality of food they will eat for the many years to come. Remember what I said in the beginning of this book? Your diet is nothing more than the food you eat. And you have to teach yourself to control the quality and quantity of your food. That's the diet the researcher is talking about. I suppose it is the hope of the researcher that the folks participating in his or her research will continue to eat the same diet after the project is completed.

Do you remember Ed from back in Chapter 7? He only wanted to lose 20 pounds and was quite happy to allow himself one full year to lose the weight. In my opinion, that's entirely too long a period and does not sufficiently challenge Ed to lose the weight.

If you look at Ed's journey in terms of calories, he could lose the 20 pounds just by cutting 800 calories from his daily food consumption. And what's 800 calories? It could be the two doughnuts he has every morning with his coffee. A doughnut is about 300 to 400 calories each. So, if Ed stops eating the doughnuts, he could shed the 20 pounds in three months (88 days). But, since this is not a journey of denial, Ed may decide he really needs his morning doughnut. So Ed can eat just one doughnut. That way he still has his doughnut (just one instead of two), and if every thing else remains the same, this one small change will result in a loss of the twenty pounds in about six months.

One pound is equal to 3400 calories. And if that doughnut is 400 calories, eating one doughnut every day will result in a gain of one pound every eight and one-half days. That's almost a pound a week! And conversely, eating one less doughnut (a 400 calorie per day reduction) could result in the loss of one pound every eight and one-half days. And to lose the twenty pounds it would take Ed only 176 days or about six months.

And if he wanted to lose more or lose the 20 pounds quicker, he could walk just one mile each day to burn 100 to 120 calories and that would result in the loss of another 13 pounds by years end. Or he could walk a golf course once a week and achieve a similar result. Or he could park his car just ½ mile from his work place and walk that distance in the morning and evening and achieve the same result. And Ed will have lost the 20 pounds long before the year's end, and will have made two very small changes in his lifestyle. And I am certain these are changes that he will find easy to continue.

And that's what this is all about. There are an unlimited number of easy and very small changes Ed could make in his lifestyle to lose the 20 pounds. But Ed has to weigh himself frequently (daily, if at all possible) to ensure he is achieving the end result at the desired rate.

And I'll say one more thing about Ed. I sure hope that the coffee and two doughnuts he is having every morning isn't his breakfast. If that constitutes his breakfast, then Ed needs to think about a more nutritious breakfast, with improved calorie versus nutrition content. But again, Ed can do this gradually. After all, it's his journey. But if he has taken my advice and has read up on these topics, his 20 pound weight loss in less than a year will be an easy and enjoyable journey, and will result not only in the desired weight loss, but improved physical health as well. And your improved health will come from not only losing weight but is also a result of your slightly increase physical activity and eating more of the foods that are good for you and less of those that are not.

I've said it before and I'll say it again, you have to do it slowly. If you make a whole slew of changes in eating and activity, you have allowed yourself to "go on a diet." You may lose some weight. But you won't keep it off because you have not slowly evolved into a healthier life style. It's that simple. And once this diet ends what then? You haven't taught yourself to live a healthier life. You haven't taught yourself how to balance the calories consumed and those burned. You've only taught yourself how to diet.

This is about eating smarter. This is about trying to reduce our calories consumed whenever possible. Let me ask you a question. If your neighbor bakes you a sheet birthday cake (rectangular and not round) with lots of icing on it (including the sides), will you eat a piece cut from the middle or will you take an edge piece or possibly a corner piece. And which of the three pieces, center, edge, or corner, contains the most calories? I'll bet that in your previous years, you would take the corner piece. Why? The corner piece tastes better. And why does the corner piece taste better. It has icing on top and on two sides. It's the sugar! And that much sugar is a waste of calories! Your priorities were in the pleasures received in eating. The consequences of the additional calories were the farthest thing from your mind. After you have been on this journey I will guarantee you will think about what you eat and will have a center piece with icing only on the top. You just cut the additional calories from the icing by two-thirds.

But, if you have been doing well, and you are well within your envelope and are confident that having an edge piece or even the corner piece will not affect your progress toward your goal, then have that piece of cake and enjoy not only the piece of cake, but also enjoy the knowledge that you can savor the cake and continue toward your goal weight. You see, it's your journey and you're in charge.

You know, I'm going to make one more comment about the wonderful doughnut to drive home the danger of a high calorie diet. And I use the word "wonderful" not in disdain. Doughnuts are wonderful: their taste is absolutely fantastic and I love doughnuts. But if you were to have two doughnuts for breakfast and have another during your coffee break, do you realize that's about 1200 calories. That's 60% of the 2000 calories the average person should consume during the entire day!

And I'll bet the fat, sugar and carbohydrate content also amount to the majority of the average person's daily limit.

And here's one more interesting fact about the human body and how weight loss can affect your journey. Do you remember I stated in an earlier chapter that it seems to be easier to lose weight at the beginning of this journey and a bit more difficult later in the journey? And do you remember I jokingly talked about tackling layers of fat? Understand first, it takes a specific number of calories for a man of 250 pounds to walk one mile. It takes fewer calories for a man of 200 pounds to walk that same one mile. The heavier you are, the more energy it takes to move. Well these two facts are related. How? If you weighed 250 pounds at the start of your journey and you walk one mile you will have expended a specific number of calories. And if you use more calories than you consume you will lose weight. But as you lose weight, say 50 pounds, you now weigh 200 pounds and will expend or use fewer calories to walk that same mile. And if your calorie consumption has remained the same, you will lose fewer pounds.

In other words, as you lose weight, you will find that you have to either increase your calories used thru activity or reduce your caloric intake. It's all about the numbers.

Chapter 20

NUTRITION AND FOOD CONTENT

In the previous chapter we talked about calories and the food elements that are the source of those calories. But there are other aspects of the food we eat that are equally important. And they could be even more important if you are someone like me who doesn't eat the proper foods. Now this should not come as a surprise, but most people who need to lose weight do not eat a well balanced diet. Some people do eat properly. And if they find they need to lose some weight, they're probably not active enough, or they are eating too much of the good things (quantity). But if you are like me, it is definitely a combination of eating and physical activity. I played sports when I was young. Baseball and tennis were the two sports I played and enjoyed. Yet, I remained overweight. And when I had problems with my spine (surgery), and could no longer play these sports, my size got completely out of hand.

There are a couple of general rules to help. Avoid, or reduce the amounts of, foods with high fat content. I suggest you try drinking and cooking with 2% or 1% milk. Avoid large amounts of salt. Everything I am saying here, you hear daily on TV. You probably know what to avoid, and what you should be eating. But remember, this is not starting out as an exercise in denial. Modifications of your eating habits should be undertaken slowly. You and your doctor should be the ones who determine what changes you want to make, should make, and believe you are committed to and able to make. But, at first, slow changes are the easiest to accomplish. More dramatic changes will come about later, but for surprisingly different reasons. We'll discuss that later.

I have only two recommendations. My first recommendation (and you should consult with your doctor on this) is to take a daily multivitamin. I did this at the insistence of my parents and doctor. And today, many years later, I still do. My second recommendation is to go to your bookstore or library and get a book on nutrition. Read it. Find out the good and bad elements of the food you presently eat. It gives you the information you need to make intelligent decisions when you decide what foods you should eats less of and what foods you could use as substitutes. Learn some things about your present diet and what changes would be helpful to an improved life. Or better yet, make an appointment and meet with a nutritionist.

You hear countless advertisements and see countless articles on fat content, calories, sugar, carbohydrates, saturated fats, unsaturated fats, trans-fats, and many other elements of our food and diet. What does all this mean? It means that we humans are beginning to be concerned about our diet. I'm not an expert on these topics and don't pretend to be. That is why I suggest you get some books on these topics, and talk to your doctor or a nutritionist about these topics and how each affects you. Generally, you should, if you're overweight, limit your fat intake. This will also reduce your calorie intake. But remember, calories are energy. We need some calories to live. And, if you just reduce your fat and calorie intake and are totally inactive, you could very well lose muscle.

And there is a second very important element to the food you eat. And that element is sugar. You can go out and find a fat free food only to discover it is loaded with sugar. And that may be even more dangerous than the fat. You will find a great debate going on about the various types of "diets" out there. Some will tell you that the amount of fat you take in is of less concern than the amount of sugar. Some will say the carbohydrates and sugar are both of major concern because the carbohydrates turn to sugar once eaten. I will tell you this. There is a major increase in the number of diabetics in those countries where the diet has evolved to consuming large amounts of sugar, and carbohydrates. There is no doubt that these elements of our diet are crucial to good health and critical in fighting the obesity and diabetes that is prevalent in these countries. You will find in this great debate there are those that will tell you that the carbohydrate free diet is not healthy because we need some carbohydrates. And they're right. You do need some carbs (carbohydrates) in your diet. The problem is we are consuming way too many carbs. You will find those that say the amount of fat we take in is of little concern; the key is to take in protein and avoid sugar and carbs. But fat is another source of calories. Therefore a diet high in fat content could also be high in calories.

You will find many sugar free foods actually have zero grams of sugar. But they contain sugar alcohols and they are high in carbohydrates. Even a diabetic could get in serious trouble eating excessive amounts of these sugar free foods.

So, they're all correct. We need to reduce the amount of fat we take in. We need to reduce the amount of sugar we take in. We need to reduce the amount of carbohydrates we take in. And now I will add my two cents worth. We also need to reduce the <u>quantity</u> of food we take in. We eat too much!

The key then is to become smarter about what you eat. Don't give up the things you like, just because they're "bad" for you. Learn to reduce your consumption of these items. Find a less "harmful" substitute. If you have cake and ice cream every night, reduce the amount. Or change to an "every other night" routine. Just try to make positive changes in your diet. Improve the "value" of what you eat, and reduce the quantity of those things you like that are of little value (other than keeping you happy). And I'm not trying to be a comedian here. If you're not happy, the chances are the attempts to lose weight, to improve your living habits will not be successful. This process MUST NOT be a miserable experience. It MUST however, be challenging and it must be something you enjoy. This following statement is the most important statement in this entire book. You must enjoy this journey. You must enjoy the results and enjoy getting those results. You must enjoy the foods you are eating (your diet). Said in a different way, you must remain comfortable with your lifestyle while working to change that lifestyle.

FAT

Ok let's talk a bit about fat. Fat is in fact, a nutrient and a source of calories. And fat is not the bad guy you have been led to believe. It's not necessarily the reason your waistline may have expanded and your cholesterol levels are high and is not necessarily the cause of anyone's poor health. But, not all fats are the same. Some are bad and some are good.

If you look at the labels on food you will see where the label states that each serving has so many calories. And it will also state the number of calories from fat. A bag of chips, for example, may state that a serving size of 12 chips contains 125 calories, and 70 calories from fat. One gram of fat supplies 9 calories. And that is twice the number of calories from carbohydrates or protein. Fat is like the other food elements in that we need some fat. Fat is necessary in that it allows the body to store vitamins A and D. There are two types of fat. There are saturated fats and unsaturated fats.

Each is used by the body in a different way and each will have a different effect on your health.   I'll discuss each a bit later.

If you eat foods high in fat content, you get large amounts of calories. If you don't burn these calories, you gain weight. Excess fat has been linked to many diseases like cancer and many diseases of the heart, such as stroke and high blood pressure. It is recommended by health experts that we should get no more that 30% of our calories from fat. If you consider those potato chips I talked about earlier, you will find that 56% of the calories were from fat. That is too high. It is clear that the fat content is too high. But it shouldn't come as a surprise that potato chips are not exactly a health food. And besides being high in fat, these chips are extremely high in carbohydrates, a source of more calories. Should you give up potato chips? No. If you like potato chips then have a few with your burger. But don't sit in front of the TV and eat a whole large bag of potato chips. And don't get caught in the trap where you say, "I only have a few chips with each meal," only to realize that you are consuming a large bag of chips each week.

How can you reduce the amount of fat you consume? Well there are really two sources of fat. The first source is the fat that is contained in the food. For example, there's fat in beef. If you love hamburger, then get lean beef. It is lower in fat content. If you find the lean beef is too dry, then grill some onions and put them in with your beef and make your own patties. Or, take the lean beef patty and place a slice of onion on top and wrap it is aluminum foil and grill it. The onion will juice it up and add some really good flavor. The second source of fat comes from the things we add to our food or put on the food. Spreads we put on our bread can contain large amounts of fat. Dressings for our salad and coverings for vegetables can contain excess amounts of fat. Milk and cheeses have large amounts of fat content. But you can use skim or low fat milk and low fat cheese. And of course there's the fat that is hidden in some foods. Many snack foods contain large amounts of fat. Doughnuts and pastries are high in fat content as are many prepared meals.

The first type of fat is called saturated fat and is found in meats and whole dairy products such as cheese, milk and cream. Too much saturated fat increases our risk of heart disease and can raise levels of cholesterol. You will also find it in many cooking oils and in some butter and margarine products, as well as many other spreads

The second fat is called unsaturated fat. This category also includes monounsaturated and polyunsaturated fats. Though this type fat does not increase the risk of heart disease, it is still not a good source of calories. Unsaturated fat can be found in vegetable oils used for cooking.

And there are trans-fats. What are they? Well, they are basically vegetable oils that have been turned into a solid fat.   They are intended to increase the shelf life of food products. Are they better? No. Just like saturated fats, they contribute to high cholesterol levels, clogged arteries, resulting in an increased chance of heart attack and stroke.

But, here's a caveat about fat. As I said, you need some fat and it is widely accepted that 30% our calories consumed should come from fat. Remember, fat is a nutrient similar to carbs and protein. Some fat is necessary for your heart health, mental health and your energy levels.

And here's another fact about fat and why we must have some fat in our diet. Do you remember the gallbladder I talked about in two previous chapters? Well, guess what. Your gallbladder depends on fat to contract and empty out its bile. Low calorie diets may not contain enough fat necessary for the gallbladder to contract normally. And that can result in gallstones. So, understanding the difference between the good and bad fats will assist you in maintaining your health during this weight loss journey.

PROTEIN

So we have talked about all the dangers of excessive amounts of some stuff in our food; fat, sugar, carbs, etc., but what about protein. Remember you need protein. Protein builds and maintains muscle. And as I mentioned earlier, we lose muscle as we age. But is widely thought the standard American diet contains too much protein. So, like all the other aspects of food, we must limit the amount of protein we consume. If we take in too much, it has to be burned as calories. And if we don't utilize all the protein, it turns to sugar – Ugh! Though I believe less carbs and less fat and higher protein will eliminate hunger later in the day, protein like everything else must be consumed in moderation. What's moderate? Read up on the subject; educate yourself or talk to your nutritionist about this.

Okay. You don't need excessive carbohydrates, excessive fat, excessive protein and excessive sugar. You need to pay attention to the content of the foods you eat. How much of these items am I consuming? There are those that will tell you it is unhealthy to totally avoid carbohydrates, and sugar, and fat. And they're right. Our problem in fighting obesity is that we don't moderate the amounts of these items. Limit your intake of those items that you know are unhealthy. Like everything else, it would be equally unhealthy if you had a diet of only meat. And, don't sit down and have a bowl of meatballs and spaghetti and consume eight pieces of bread with lots of margarine spread all over it. Have a little less spaghetti and only one piece of bread and limit the butter. Notice I said butter. Why? Avoid the trans-fats. In other words, when it comes to eating, you need to "get smart."

If, as I propose, you become more aware of the food you eat, paying attention to the labels on that food, and watch the effects of that food and the quantities of that food (daily weighing) you will also soon find that you are consuming less fat than before you began this journey. I can guarantee you I now consume more protein and less sugar, less carbohydrates, and less fat than I did before I started this journey.

In essence, what it comes down to is this. Read the labels and be aware of what you are consuming. And again, you don't have to go crazy trying to find the low fat, low sugar, low carb, low calorie food that is the answer to your prayers. It doesn't exist. And if you did find it, I can guarantee it will taste absolutely horrible. And you will be miserable if you force yourself to eat it. Just try to be a little more selective and take it slowly and try different things and see what works for you.

Here's one final statement about food. And this really sums up my position on the food I eat, considering both quantity and quality. Yes we should avoid fatty foods. And yes, I often have bacon with my eggs for breakfast. And yes bacon is high is saturated fat. So, am I talking out of both sides of my mouth? Absolutely not. You see I love bacon. But I have only one slice. Again moderation is the key. You don't have to completely give up the things you love. Just moderate your consumption of these items. I guarantee the nutritional factors of my two eggs and one strip of bacon is far better than that of a cup of coffee and two doughnuts or a bowl of cereal loaded with sugar and high fat content milk. I can also guarantee I won't be hungry and looking for a vending machine around 10:30 AM.

Let me ask you a question. Are you surprised that we should not be consuming excessive amounts of the various elements of the food we eat? That's what we have been told for years. It's been advised for years that we need a balanced diet. And as you move along this journey, I believe you will begin to move toward a balanced diet. It is not unusual for those of us who are overweight to realize that our diet is not balanced. The vast majority of us have gotten in our present condition by consuming too much of the foods that are not good for us. We have an "unbalanced" diet. And as you make the various changes in your diet, reducing the amounts of the bad food (notice I did not say eliminate) and replacing them with better choices, you will be moving toward a better balance in the foods you eat. And that alone will result in a major reduction in the calories you consume.

Folks, I keep saying this over and over. It's about moderation. It's about eating smart and avoiding excesses of those items that have high concentrations of fat, sugar, carbohydrates, etc.

Chapter 21
MEALS, SNACKS AND OTHER IDEAS

Well, we have talked about a lot of issues. We've covered the importance of knowing what is in the various foods we eat. We've talked about calories and that through selective eating and activity we will need to burn more calories than we consume in order to lose weight. And we will need to achieve a balance of these calories to maintain a healthy weight. We've talked about the fat, carbohydrates, sugar and other elements of foods. We have established a goal weight and have created a graph. Our envelope is set at just the right slope (rate). The attitude is right and the commitment is there. So we're ready to fly. Correct? Absolutely yes!

So, what's this chapter about? Well, think of this as a primer. It is nothing more than some thoughts and experiences on meals, food selection, snacking and a few other ideas about selective eating and some thoughts as well about various activities you may find helpful. Some of these ideas may help you start thinking about ways you can eat smarter and maybe find some special and enjoyable activities for you to burn calories. And I'm going to repeat myself one more time. Remember, you don't have to avoid the foods you love. Just limit how often you eat them. And when you do eat them, reduce or limit how much you eat.

I will share one bit of info with you. I have found that limiting carbohydrates is a good method of avoiding hunger. And I suggest you try this experiment. Have two eggs for breakfast one morning. This is a high protein, low carbohydrate meal. Do not have any toast or biscuits or orange juice. Avoid the carbs. You could, if you want, have one or two strips of bacon. Then see if you have any hunger pains around 10:30 or prior to eating lunch. The next morning have a bowl of cereal with milk. And, you should watch for any signs of hunger around 10:30 or prior to eating your lunch. I have found that a low carb high protein meal reduces the need to snack because there are less hunger pains. And if you do have hunger pains, satisfy that hunger with a snack of peanuts, or walnuts. That's a high protein, low carbohydrate, zero sugar snack.

You may also find that having a couple of low carb high protein meals will help you get off of a plateau and start a downward trend again. You may also find that limiting your carbs is a good way to ensure your "start" period is not too long. Now understand that I am not endorsing the eating of carbohydrate free foods. We all need some carbs. But eating a big bowl of pasta at every meal and sitting and watching TV all day long are a sure fire way to an overweight condition and poor health.

And again, please remember that you don't have to avoid the foods you love. Just limit how often you eat them. And when you do eat them, limit how much you eat. Let's take a look at four items; breakfast, lunch, dinner, and snacks.

Breakfast is the start of your day and a good place to start. I'll start with a rare comment about the one food I suggest you avoid. And that food item is the ever present doughnut. Why? Well, it's high in sugar, fat, and carbohydrates. And there is very little about the doughnut that is good, except of course, the taste. Does that mean you can never have a doughnut? No! You can have anything you want. The question is how bad do you want it? And there is nothing wrong with having a doughnut on occasion. But if you have two or three every morning for breakfast, you have a problem. Of course, you could be skinny as a rail and lead a very active lifestyle. In that case you can have your doughnuts. If that describes you, my only question is, why are you reading this book? I'll share one additional comment about the doughnut. I once attended a seminar at a local hospital where the presenter referred to the doughnut as a "heart grenade." And that sums up my opinion about the doughnut. Does that mean I never eat doughnuts? No. In fact I had one just this week. But I don't eat three or four a day as I once did. I may go a month or two before having another one. And if I'm trying to shed a few pounds or I'm on a plateau, you can bet I won't eat a doughnut.

What should you have for breakfast? Again, remember you are trying to reduce your sugar intake, minimize the carbohydrates to help in losing weight, and maximize the protein to avoid hunger pains. You could have cereal with skim, 1%, or 2% milk. But remember most cereals and the milk are high in carbs. You could have a bowl of oatmeal. You could have some bacon and eggs. And what should you do about bread products? Do you have to have biscuits or toast with your eggs? Well, if you have to have some toast, have a piece (or half a piece) of whole wheat toast. Or you may decide to have half a biscuit. And in a couple of weeks when you hit a plateau you may decide to no longer have the biscuit. Or just have half of a biscuit ever once in a while. And limit the butter (you put on the toast or biscuit). And what about pancakes? Well, there are some low carb pancakes out there and there is nothing wrong with having these delicious items on occasion. And by the way they are very good. And coming from me that's a complement. There is also an oatmeal pancake that tastes very good. But don't smother them with three cups of syrup that contain a two day supply of sugar. By the way, there are a couple of sugar free syrups that are absolutely wonderful. And speaking of sugar, if you have the cereal, make absolutely certain you select a serial low in sugar. If you must have a cereal high in sugar have a bit less. And if you always add sugar, add less. In fact, you really should try to avoid adding sugar to your cereal. Try a different cereal. Adding pure sugar to cereal is a really bad habit. Try your best to avoid it.

And what about fruit? There's nothing wrong with putting some fruit on your cereal, or just having a bowl of fruit for breakfast. Okay. So the fruit has the natural sugars and maybe some carbs. But isn't a bowl of fruit and a glass of orange juice better for you (in terms of fat and calories) than six giant pancakes and three cups of sugar laden syrup? I will guarantee you the pancake breakfast contains six times as many calories as the fruit breakfast. And I will also guarantee you two things. First, when you move away from the table, you will be much more uncomfortable after eating the pancake breakfast. And second, by 11:00 AM you will be hungry and searching for a snack if you had the pancake breakfast. And you may also find the same thing happens if you have the fruit breakfast. This whole process is all about choices. Either you choose to eat smart and get healthy or you choose to ignore your condition and take your chances with poor health and gamble you can live many more years carrying the extra weight. And if you don't like fruit and just love the pancakes, eat them less frequently and instead of eating six, try eating three. I can almost guarantee you have been eating twice as much as you need and you don't even realize it. And get the better pancakes and the sugar free syrup.

Lunch is really no different that breakfast. The name of the game is to eat smarter. You have to make smarter choices. If you choose to continue to eat the things you love, and you know they are of less nutritional value, you have to eat smaller servings. But even in eating the things you love, you can still make some intelligent choices. As I stated earlier, when I have a bacon cheeseburger I will either remove the top half of the bun or sometimes remove both halves of the bun and just eat the meat and cheese. In the vast majority of cases, the bun doesn't taste all that good anyway. The bun is really nothing more than a tool used to pick up the burger and eat it without getting your fingers all greasy. It doesn't really add that much to the taste. And yes I will sometimes even have the french fries. But I may eat just a few. Or, sometimes I'll skip the fries and have onion rings. A bowl of soup is another smart choice. Many times, I will have a couple of hard boiled eggs. If I'm able to fix my lunch, I microwave some meatballs and swiss cheese. Again, I place the emphasis on minimizing the sugar and carbohydrates I consume, and ensure the protein is there. And if you like those tiny square hamburgers, you can order two, and throw away both top halves of the buns and combine then to have a double meat burger. In the case of these little burgers, that steamed bun really does add to the taste. But I am still able to halve the amount of white bread (and carbs) I consume.

If you like salads, that's great. Just be careful of the various dressings. Some contain vast amounts of fat, sugar and carbohydrates. If you have a full meal for lunch, again, be selective and avoid the high sugar, high carbohydrate foods. If you have the choice, baked and broiled is far better that fried. But if you're like me and like only fried food, then you have to make your choices elsewhere. And, as was the case with breakfast, try reducing the amount of food you eat for lunch. I can almost guarantee you will find you have been consuming more food than you require.

One thing you might try is to define one meal as the "light" meal for the day. Though this can be of value, you must be aware that having a light meal can have some negative aspects. If for example, you have a light lunch, and find yourself needing a snack at 3:00 PM, and the quality of snack food available is not ideal, you could be making a mistake. Let's say you usually have eight meatballs covered with provolone cheese. But today you decide to eat a light lunch and have a small cup of vegetable soup. Then at three o'clock you're hungry and the vending machine at work only offers candy bars or a bag of chips. The snack resulted in losing the gains you hoped to achieve with the light lunch. Again, there is no rule that you have to have a light lunch. It is a choice you can make if you know it works for you. You may decide to try this to compensate for a big meal at the awards dinner you attended last night. Or maybe you have a light lunch on Thursday and Friday or on Monday and Tuesday to compensate for the "weakend." If you do decide to have an occasional light lunch or breakfast, make sure you have some quality snack food available, if you need it. You may find that after several weeks of having light meals you don't need the snack. If that's the case, then you have just proven to yourself that for years you have been eating too much food at meal time. After all, if you have a light lunch and don't get hungry, then it is evident that the amount of food at those meals is sufficient. And as an added bonus, you should find that your weight starts to decrease. Oh how you will be amazed at what you will learn about yourself and your "old" habits.

If you do decide to try having a light meal, I strongly suggest it be high in protein and low in sugar and carbs. In that way, you will minimize your chances of getting hungry later in the day.

And speaking of light meals, you may have noticed I mentioned only lunch and breakfast when talking about light meals. The reason is rather simple. The amount of time between meals is greatest between dinner and breakfast. On average, the amount of time between breakfast and lunch and between lunch and dinner is 6 hours or less. The time between dinner and breakfast averages 12 hours. Of course, this is another reason people snack in the evening. Because of the length of time between dinner and breakfast, it is important that your dinner provide sufficient energy and nutrition to get you through to tomorrow's breakfast. Again, it is better to provide your needs at a meal rather than rely on snacking, only because we tend to snack on those foods that are less than ideal. But if you have snacks that are good quality food, there is nothing wrong with experimenting with light meals and snacking on these good quality foods.

It is no surprise to learn that dinner is no different than the other meals of the day. Again, be selective. Avoid or limit the amount of those foods that are high in fat, sugar and carbohydrates. Emphasize the food items high in protein and avoid or limit the quantities of the items high in sugar and carbohydrates. When deciding to have a light dinner, be mindful that breakfast may be 12 hours away. I would suggest that you have a light dinner only to compensate for an unusually large lunch. And if you have a light dinner, ensure the availability of good quality snack food should the need arise in the evening. Again, you can be creative.

In my case, I decided that I would make most of my eating modifications in my breakfast and lunch meals and my snacking habits. I decided not to modify my dinner meal. Later on, when I found the need to make some additional changes to stay inside my envelope, I began to evaluate my dinner meals. It is there that I discovered I was eating far more than I needed. As I have stated time and again, it is all about making many small changes that makes this system work. Major changes are difficult to endure.

And one last comment about dinner and the hours afterward. There in no reason in the world you can't go to bed just a wee bit hungry. In fact, many people discover that they have been snacking in the evening not because they were hungry, but because they don't want to wake up in the morning hungry. We often snack in the evening out of habit and not because of hunger pains. There were times I had a peanut butter snack and had difficulty in sleeping because of the quantity of peanut butter in my stomach. And I would wake up with indigestion. And the very next night I would make the same mistake again. Why? We often snack because we are creatures of habit. It could take a really concerted effort, as was my case, to stop snacking in the evening.

Let's talk more about snacking. If you are like me, you love to snack. Put me in front of the TV with a spoon and a jar of peanut butter and I'm in heaven. Even though peanut butter is very high in protein, it is equally high in fat and loaded with sugar and therefore calories. But I couldn't survive without it. And I mean that in all sincerity. I love the stuff and can't imagine living without it. But I had to learn to eat it in moderation. And there were times that I stopped eating it altogether to ensure my rate of weight loss continued. And it wasn't a difficult decision. As much as I love peanut butter, I loved what I was becoming even more and I wasn't about to jeopardize it by "pigging out" with the jar of peanut butter and a spoon.

Snacking is a necessary evil. And if your are like me and usually snack on those items that are high in sugar, fat, calories, etc, then you have to avoid the snack, or reduce the amount of these items you snack on. Again, be selective. Snack on fruits. I was 29 years old and re-discovered that red thing called the apple. And I must re-emphasize the comment I made about avoiding snacks. It can be done. The key for me was to emphasize the protein in my meals. But don't fall into the trap that you can concentrate on protein and ignore the fat, sugar, carbs, etc. You must also do what you can to minimize those elements in your food.

You will find, as I did, that after a certain amount of time, and it's impossible to say how long, your stomach will actually shrink in size. You will find that it takes less quantity of food to satisfy you. But until this wonderful miracle occurs, go ahead and snack on those foods that are low in calories (fruits), or snack on your favorites, but limit the quantity. There are many, many low calorie snack foods in your supermarket.

What you will find is that at some point in time, you will hit a plateau. And after trying several things to get started on a downward slope again, you'll try not snacking. And eventually there will be nights when you will forget to have your snack. You will be amazed the way your lifestyle will slowly change. Sometimes this change will occur without your even being aware of it. I know many of us snack not because were hungry, but because we have been snacking for years, hungry or not. We are creatures of habit.

There is only one rule, or piece of advice that I will give. And really, I shouldn't use the word rule. The use of that word sort of implies that this piece of advice is an absolute must. And it is not. It is only a suggestion. You should try to avoid eating after 8 PM. The body does not digest food well, when sleeping. I believe we have all had a very late dinner and gone right to bed, only to wake up in the middle of the night or the next morning wishing we hadn't eaten so much or so late. If this happens to you, watch your weight on your graph. Chances are pretty good that this will put you on a plateau. And it may take a couple of days to get started on a downward slope again. My advice then is to avoid late dinners, and late night snacking.

If you decide you don't want to avoid late night snacking, that's okay. After all, this is a process where you determine what it takes to stay inside your envelope. But, if you find yourself on a plateau, or going outside (above) your envelope, try to limit or stop your late night snacking and see if it doesn't help.

Do you remember we talked earlier about the positive aspects of sleep? Here's another one. It should not come as a surprise that if you stay up late, there is an increased chance you will need a snack. So if you're on a plateau or trying to increase your weight loss rate and snacking is a problem, go to bed earlier. In essence, you're avoiding the temptation.

What are some other good snack materials? A hard boiled egg can be a great snack. Peanuts, cashews or walnuts can be a great snack, high in protein and practically no carbs or sugar. I like to take a thin slice of bologna and wrap it around a mozzarella cheese stick. And if you decide that bologna is not exactly your idea of a health food, try your cheese stick with a slice of lean boiled ham. Celery sticks and peanut butter also make for a good snack. Pork rinds can be a good snack since they contain no carbs, no sugar and are high in protein. Now I know that some of these items are also high in fat. And though I tend to not place much emphasis on the fat, it is only because the sugar and carbohydrates are more influential on the balance between food intake (calories consumed) and activity (calories burned). And I'm talking about having just a few of these chips or pork rinds for a snack. I'm not proposing you eat a whole bag of these for a snack. Again, limit the size of your snack. I can almost guarantee that when you snack, you do so out of habit and not because of any enormous hunger pain. So, if snacking is essential, to satisfy hunger or to appease the habit of snacking, then limit the size of the snack. I would never propose that anyone eat bags and bags of pork rinds, or live on bologna and cheese. A steady diet of any of these foods is not a good lifestyle. A high fat diet can be as dangerous as a high sugar diet.   They both result in your taking in an excess of calories.

If, as I propose, you become more aware of the food you eat, paying attention to the labels on that food, and watching the effect of that food (type and quantity) on your weight (daily weighing), you will find you are consuming less fat than before you began this journey. Yes, I have some peanuts or pork rinds very often. But I can guarantee you I now consume more protein and less sugar, less carbohydrates and less fat than I did before I started my journey. This is the exact point that was made in discussing all the other diets. When you start thinking and paying attention to what you eat. You will lose weight no matter what dieting process you undertake, provided you have made a commitment and have a good attitude toward your effort.

In essence, what it comes down to is this. Read the labels and be aware of what you are eating. And again, you don't have to go crazy trying to find the low fat, low carb, low sugar, low calorie food that is the answer to your prayers. It doesn't exist. And if you did find it, I can guarantee it will taste absolutely horrible. And you will be miserable if you force yourself to eat it.

Now let's talk a bit about various ways of burning calories. And once again, don't think about various exercise routines that you might start. This is not about joining a health club. Of course if you already have a membership at a health club and "working out" is part of your daily routine, then that's great and you should continue. In your case, you probably need to emphasize the eating side of the equation. Or increase the number of visits or increase the level of the existing exercise routines. Or, increase your other activities.

But most of us don't have health club memberships and since that is not part of our daily life, running out and joining a health club is not, in my opinion, the answer. What is the answer? Well, I suggest you first think about your existing daily activities and schedules, and where you might make some changes. For example, when you arrive at work, is it your primary goal to park as close as possible to your office building. Why? Could you park a couple of blocks away and walk? And when you arrive at work, do you always take the elevator? What's wrong with taking the stairs? Okay. Your brief case is heavy and you don't want to perspire and get your shirt or blouse all wet. So take the elevator up and use the stairs when you go down to the first floor for lunch and at the end of the day. And after lunch take a short walk. Even a walk around the block does wonders for you in more ways that you can imagine. First, this leisure walk burns calories that you wouldn't ordinarily burn reading the newspaper. Second, it brings about awareness that you are serious about this journey. And when you head toward the vending machine at three o'clock, the memory of that short walk around the block will be in your head and will have a major influence on the food you select for your snack. And if you have a meeting across town, take a cab and walk the last two blocks. There are all kinds of activities that will help to burn calories. And guess what! This type of activity can reduce the stress levels of your job.

And what about your evenings at home? Are their any opportunities to burn some extra calories there? You bet there are. You just have to discover them and take the opportunity when it presents itself. A short walk or a short bike ride can be fun besides burning calories. And on weekends a walk or bike ride in the park or on the beach can easily become something you look forward to. And when you go to the store, you don't have to park as close to the entrance as possible. Take the opportunity to walk a bit. And if you drive to the mall don't park near the store where you intend to shop. Park at the other end of the mall and enjoy the walk. And, as you know, though I don't like the word exercise, there are a few routines you can do in your bed before you go to sleep that can not only burn calories, but also firm up your stomach muscles. And if you are able, you might consider swimming or taking up tennis. But again, the various activities that you select to increase the rate at which you burn calories must be something you are dedicated to or something you enjoy. And who knows, you may even enjoy tennis after a while.

If the various activities are not something you enjoy, then they will become, or already are, a burden. The activities you perform must become second nature. You must perform these activities because that is you and not because you "have to burn some calories." If it doesn't become a way of life for you, then when you get to the desired weight, you'll probably stop the activity and gain the weight back.

So, you see this whole process is about choices and the results of those choices. And these are choices you decide you want to make and choices that you know you can make and will live with for many years to come.

My only other suggestion is that you take some time to sit down and really think about the lifestyle choices that you could make. In fact, I suggest you get a notebook and record all these ideas. And when recording these ideas, don't just write down "eat less." Be specific and write "eat less mashed potatoes. " Or, you could write "stop eating french fries at lunch time," or "eat only the bottom half of hamburger bun." And the same thing goes for ways to burn calories. You could write down, for example, take a 15 minute walk on Tuesdays and Thursdays. And each time you think of something else you might be able to do, write it down. And as I said before, you don't have to make all the changes at once. Do them in stages and see the results of each lifestyle change. And record the date you undertake each change in lifestyle. At some point I guarantee you will go back and look at your graph and look at the dates of the various changes you made and relate your successes with those changes. There will come a point in time when you hit a plateau you will be glad you can go back to your notes and pick up on an idea that might help in getting off the plateau or back inside your envelope. And you might even find that the results of your Tuesday and Thursday walks were so successful, that adding Saturday and Sunday might be just the thing to get you back in inside your envelope and get back to losing pounds.

Now I know that you may be thinking that this is becoming a lot of work. But remember, when you work with this notebook, it helps to keep your awareness tuned in to the fact that you are working on lifestyle changes. There will be times you will order lunch and completely forget and just dive into that pile of french fries. But if you do things that heighten your awareness of your lifestyle changes and keep you tuned in, your "old habits" won't hurt you as often.

And here's one more bit of information that could prove interesting to your journey and actually assist you in the process of food selection. Make a concerted effort to be aware of when you become hungry. Then go back and examine what you had to eat at your last meal (or last snack). And also make a concerted effort to be aware that you, for example, did not get hungry between today's lunch and dinner. Then go back and examine what you had for lunch. Was your lack of hunger due to a high protein lunch or did you eat more than your normal amount of food? These are little tidbits of information or realizations that you can watch for that can help you along this journey. As I related before, I was amazed that after a breakfast of two eggs and one slice of bacon, I did not have hunger pains around 10:30. But if I had a bowl of low sugar cereal and 1% milk, there's a good chance I would find myself hungry at 10:30. Now this may not be the case during your journey. But watch for these types of things. Be aware of what you eat (both quality and quantity) and how it affects the rest of your day. Like I keep saying, this is a learning experience. Be aware of what's going on and learn from it.

Chapter 22

RE-START

I talked in previous chapters about the slope of the graph. If it is too steep, you may have over challenged yourself and if it is not steep enough, you may not have challenged yourself sufficiently. Here I'd like to delve a bit deeper in these two situations and what to do if at some point in time during this journey, you decide that one of the above conditions exists. Either you have over-challenged yourself or you decide you can do better and wish you had set a higher weight loss goal, or stated differently, wish you had decided to lose the weight at a bit faster rate.

First of all, this problem usually occurs during the first month or two of the journey. But, be careful. As you will read later, it is best to not modify your graphs during the first two or three months because things can and probably will change. I strongly suggest you wait until you are well into your journey, say the fourth month, before you decide to modify your rate of weight loss. Most often the mistake is that we set too high a weight loss rate. And this is a very common mistake. We all think, because of our enthusiasm, our commitment and our can-do attitude that we will lose weight at a rate that is a bit unrealistic. If you lose weight in the first three or four weeks at a good rate and then the weight lost per week begins to slow down and you just can't get back in the envelope you run the risk of losing your enthusiasm and ending your journey of discovery and better health. If that's the case, just re-calculate your weight loss over a longer period of time and lose the weight at a bit slower rate. Re-draw your graph with your two goal lines at a not-so-steep decline. But do not change your loss rate more than once. Changing your rate multiple times can be the result of a poor attitude or a lack of commitment.

Here's an example. Stephen weighs 220 pounds and wants to weigh 175 pounds. That means he wants to lose 45 pounds. He decides he can lose it over 6 months. Now that's a bit rapid, but he thinks he can do it. So his desired weight loss rate is about 7 and ½ pounds per month or about 1 and ¾ pounds per week. Stephen draws his graphs and begins his journey. In the first week he loses nothing. That's normal. But then the pounds start to disappear. In the second week he loses 2 pounds. And in the third week he loses 3 pounds and in the fourth week he loses another 3 pounds. Okay. So far he has lost 8 pounds over four weeks. That means he is losing weight at a faster rate than desired. His desired weight loss rate is 7 pounds in four weeks and he has lost 8 pounds. He is happy and is below his upper goal line. But then over the next month he loses only an additional 5 pounds instead of the 7 and ½ pounds desired. He tries, but can't increase the weight loss rate without making dietary changes he is uncomfortable with or maybe he doesn't have the time to devote to any increased physical activity.

Stephen has to make a choice. He can either give up and end his journey and be happy he lost 8 pounds or he can suck it up and make the additional changes needed. But if he has problems with these needed additional changes, then his attitude and commitment will suffer and the chances of failing to end his journey at his desired weight are increasing. But he has a third choice. And, in fact, it may be the best choice.

All Stephen has to do is recalculate his weight loss rate and redraw his graphs to accommodate his more realistic weight loss rate. He wants to weigh 175 pounds. So instead of setting his goal date out 6 months, he can do it in 9 months or about 39 weeks and his weight loss rate will be about 1.15

pounds per week or about 5 pounds per month. Who cares if it takes 9 months instead of 6? Slower is better anyway. And a slow method of changing one's lifestyle has a better chance of continuation of the new lifestyle after the weight has been lost. And it makes Stephen's journey more pleasant. It's the end that counts and not how long it took to get there. And what Stephen could do is draw his lower goal line (the bottom of the envelope) at the old rate of 7 and ½ pounds per month. Then draw a new upper goal line at less steep slope of say 5 pounds per month. That way he would have both his old rate and new rate shown on his graph.

The other possibility of wanting to redraw your graph is a bit more complicated. And the complication is not in re-drawing the graph, but the repercussions of the decision to lose weight at possibly too fast a rate. Let's say that Stephen, as in the above case, losses 8 pounds the first month. But let's say that he losses another 8 pounds the second month. He realizes that if he continues to lose 8 pounds a month, he can lose the whole 45 pounds in just over 5 and ½ months. Well, as in the above case, Stephen can redraw his graph to average his weight loss over the 5 and ½ months or about 24 weeks. His weight loss rate will be about 1.875 pounds per week and about 8.2 pounds per month.

I said that this second graph change is a bit more complicated. The complication isn't about redrawing the graph. That part's simple. The complication deals with the long term results of deciding to lose the weight at a faster rate. First, there's the medical side of this issue. As I said earlier, losing weight at too rapid a rate can be detrimental to your health. If this rapid weight loss is due to Stephen starving himself, then it's a very dangerous and bad decision. If the rapid weight loss is due to Stephen's discovery that he just loves taking an evening bike ride and loves to take a quick 15 minute walk everyday after lunch, then that's great.

But that brings us to the second negative side of Stephen's decision to lose the weight at a more rapid rate. Is this new lifestyle something that Stephen will continue after his journey is completed. Will he continue to starve himself? Probably not. And in this case he will, in all probability, re-gain the weight. Stephen didn't develop a new lifestyle he can live with for the rest of his life. He allowed the journey to turn into a "diet."

And what if his dietary changes are minor or not at all, but his weight loss is the result of his new found love of cycling and walking. That's great and he will probably have a very successful journey to his desired weight. But I suggest Stephen place this book on his book shelf. Because someday, he is going to get older and find he is unable to perform at his current level. And when this happens, he is going to be forced to make dietary changes to compensate for his decreased level of activity. Here's that balance between calories consumed versus calories burned. He may very well need to read this book again in later life.

Do I make the decision to redraw my graph? Be careful here. And to make my point, go back and look at my graphs for January, February and March. In January, it looks as though I should have decided to lose weight at a faster rate. If I had redrawn my graph at the end of January, it would have been a huge mistake. In February the desired weight loss rate and the actual weight loss rate were very close. Then in March it looked like my desired weight loss rate was greater than I could accomplish. I could have redrawn my graphs then. But again, it would have been a big mistake. If I had redrawn my graphs to better match my weight loss rate in March, I would have extended the journey out to over a year. The answer in March was to "meet the challenge" and do more lifestyle modifications to lose weight at my desired rate and not redraw the chart at a reduced rate.

To repeat, my advice is to not modify your graph during the first three months. And here's the reason. The first month is the start and beginning periods and weight loss rate will fluctuate a great deal. During this first month, you're just getting started. Don't be too quick to modify things. The second month you will probably lose more than expected. Again, don't be too quick to modify your graph. You're just getting started to lose weight. The third month is where you might want to consider modifying your graph if you are continuing to lose weight at a faster or slower rate than desired.

WARNING

Don't let a series of plateaus or a decreased weight loss rate convince you that it's easier to redraw your graph rather than make some decisions to modify poor eating habits or to increase your activities. If you modify the graph rather than modify these poor lifestyle habits, you could be falling into realm of "It's easier to reduce my goal than to work hard." But remember, that choice is yours.

Chapter 23

IN CONCLUSION

Do you remember in grade school when you had to write a speech and stand before your classmates and give the speech or had to debate one side of a particular issue? Do you also remember that you always ended it with the phrase "In conclusion?" And that's where you re-emphasized all the points you intended to make during your speech. You were absolutely certain that you needed to use an "in conclusion" section in your talk because you know you just had to make absolutely certain your fellow classmates got the important points and so you stated all those important points one more time.

And do you also remember that your teacher told you to remove the "in conclusion" section of your speech and instead ensure you emphasized and clearly stated your points during the body of your presentation?

Well, I don't really need an "in conclusion" chapter to this book. Do I? You're probably sick and tired of hearing that you need to take it slow, that you need to make small changes (one at a time), and that you're developing a lifestyle you can live with for years to come. And do you remember how many times you read the phrase "just eat less of it." It reminds me of the old phrase, "You're beating a dead horse." Yes, I have beaten that horse enough. But I have repeated it many times because it is the **essence** of this journey.

There's one more point I'd like to make. I am sure that in the beginning chapters of this book you considered this process as something you could very possibly accomplish. Then in later chapters, when you started hearing about calories and reading labels and keeping notebooks and all the other hints I put forward, you began thinking this is too much like work. I don't want to do all this! If that sounds like you, then put all that aside for now, and just concentrate on your graph and some lifestyle modifications. Don't even think of all the other "stuff" (recommendations) that I proposed. Later, when your successes are hindered by plateaus, you might then consider some of the other recommendations and hints.

So, you're right. There's no need to talk about all these points anymore. You have heard it enough! So I'll not talk about any of them, with one exception. And that concerns the importance of enjoying this journey you are about to take. Diets, for the most part are not enjoyable experiences; other than the enjoyment of seeing pounds disappear. But you must make this an enjoyable experience. And in doing that you must not disrupt your existing life with any dieting requirements. The changes you make must fit right in with your existing lifestyle and modify it only in tiny bits and pieces. The smaller the changes, the longer your journey must be. And a longer journey is okay. It's up to you as to how long to make the journey and therefore how large are the lifestyle changes to be.

Believe me, it can be an enjoyable experience for three specific reasons.

1. It's easy to make small changes whether they pertain to the food you eat or the activities you undertake.
2. You don't have to give up the foods you love. You just - - Oops, I almost said it again. But you know what I mean.
3. You will love what is happening to your body, your self-esteem, and more importantly, your health.

So, in conclusion, I'll only say … Enjoy your journey.